High Protein, Diabetic-Friendly Vegan Pregnancy Cookbook For First Time Moms

Optimized Vegan Solutions With Delicious, Easy-to-follow Recipes For Pregnant Women Managing Diabetes

By
Bertha Seward

Copyright

About the Author

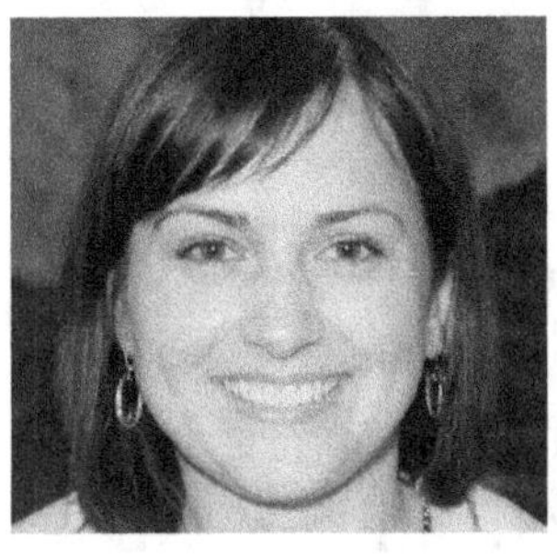 Bertha Seward is a passionate and dedicated author. She is a holistic health coach, and advocate for plant-based living. With years of research in the field of nutrition and a deep understanding of the unique nutritional needs of pregnant women, Bertha brings a wealth of expertise and insight to her work. Her journey into the world of veganism began as a personal quest for better health and vitality, but it was her own experience with pregnancy that ignited her passion for supporting other vegan moms-to-be.

Driven by a desire to empower women to embrace the benefits of a plant-based diet during pregnancy, Bertha embarked on a mission to create a comprehensive resource that would provide expectant mothers with the knowledge, guidance, and recipes they need to thrive throughout pregnancy and beyond. But beyond her expertise in nutrition, Bertha's warmth, compassion, and genuine desire to support mothers shines through in every page of her book. She understands the challenges and joys of pregnancy firsthand and approaches her work with empathy, understanding, and a deep commitment to helping women embrace the transformative journey of motherhood with confidence and vitality.

As a mother, Bertha is uniquely positioned to offer guidance and support to expectant mothers navigating the complexities of pregnancy while maintaining a vegan lifestyle. With her book, she hopes to inspire and empower women to nourish their bodies, support their babies' development, and embrace the incredible journey of pregnancy and motherhood with grace and gratitude.

Table Of Contents

Introduction

A journey of beauty and transformation, pregnancy is a time of expectation, joy, and the promise of fresh beginnings. You are obviously excited to provide yourself and your developing child the finest care possible as a first-time mother starting this amazing journey.

It may be quite difficult to navigate the world of pregnancy nutrition, particularly for those who are vegan or have diabetes. This book is your all-inclusive guide to adopting a high-protein, vegan diet that is suitable for people with diabetes during pregnancy, guaranteeing the best possible health and wellbeing for you and your unborn child.

These sections provide a plethora of knowledge, useful advice, and mouthwatering dishes that will satisfy your gastronomic desires and nutritional requirements during this unique period. This book is your go-to resource if you need advice on controlling blood sugar levels, balancing macronutrients, or just getting creative in the kitchen.

We've put together a selection of healthful, tasty recipes that highlight the abundance of plant-based ingredients and satisfy the particular dietary needs of expectant mothers, all while drawing on the most recent research in nutrition and pregnancy health, as well as the knowledge of medical professionals and seasoned mothers.

Every meal, from filling snacks to decadent desserts, from healthy breakfasts to substantial dinners, is carefully designed to provide vital nutrients, support stable blood sugar levels, and satiate your palate without sacrificing flavor or variety.

A vital macronutrient for tissue development and repair, including the growing baby's tissues, is protein. To satisfy their increased nutritional needs, pregnant women—especially those who follow a vegan diet—must prioritize foods high in protein.

The need to control blood sugar levels is increased during pregnancy, especially for diabetic women. Expectant moms may maximize glycemic management and provide themselves and their newborns with optimum nutrition by embracing a vegan diet that is favorable to diabetics.

Carbs and lipids, in addition to protein, are essential for maintaining energy levels and promoting general health throughout pregnancy. In order to provide appropriate nutrition, stabilize blood sugar, and encourage satiety, it is essential to understand how to balance these macronutrients.

It's important to pay attention to the intake of micronutrients in addition to macronutrients. Pregnancy health depends on key nutrients including iron, calcium, omega-3 fatty acids, vitamin B12, folate, zinc, and vitamin D. These nutrients should be addressed via thoughtful meal choices and supplementation as needed.

Particularly when it comes to controlling their diabetes, many expectant mothers are worried about how they will be able to satisfy their nutritional demands while following a vegan diet. This section answers frequently asked questions and offers helpful advice for resolving dietary obstacles.

Chapter 1

Understanding the Basics of Vegan Nutrition During Pregnancy

Increased dietary requirements occur during pregnancy because the body is working extra hard to support the fetus's growth and development while also keeping the mother healthy. Making sure that women who follow a vegan diet are getting enough of these vital minerals becomes critical.

- **Macronutrients in Vegan Pregnancy Nutrition**

Protein

- **Importance:** Protein promotes the growth of maternal tissue and is necessary for the development and repair of all tissues, including those of the growing fetus.

- **Food Sources:** Edamame, seitan, beans, lentils, chickpeas, tofu, tempeh, quinoa, nuts, seeds, and whole grains are vegan sources of protein.

- **Consideration:** To make sure they are receiving all the required amino acids, pregnant women should try to incorporate a range of foods high in protein in their diet. It's also critical to consistently eat meals high in protein to support your body's increased protein demands throughout pregnancy.

Carbohydrates

- **Importance:** The body uses carbohydrates as its main energy source to power both the growing fetus and the mother.

- **Food Sources:** Whole grains (brown rice, quinoa, oats, barley), starchy vegetables (sweet potatoes, potatoes, maize), legumes (beans, lentils, chickpeas), fruits, and some vegetables (carrots, beets) are vegan sources of carbs.

- **Consideration:** Opt for complex carbs instead of refined ones since they are higher in nutrients and fiber. To guarantee a well-rounded diet, include a range of carbohydrate sources in your meals and snacks.

Fat

- **Importance:** During pregnancy, hormone synthesis, brain development, and nutrition absorption all depend on healthy fats.

- **Food Sources:** Avocados, almonds, walnuts, pistachios, avocado oil, flaxseeds, hemp seeds, olives, coconut, and plant-based oils including olive, avocado, and coconut oil are vegan sources of good fats.

- **Consideration:** Give unsaturated fats—such as mono- and polyunsaturated fats—priority as they are good for the heart. Avoid trans fats and restrict your consumption of saturated fats since they may be harmful to your health.

- **Essential Micronutrients for a Vegan Pregnancy**

Iron

- **Importance:** During pregnancy, iron is essential for the synthesis of red blood cells and the prevention of anemia.
- **Food Sources:** Legumes, beans, tofu, tempeh, quinoa, dried fruits (apricots, raisins), lentils, cereals fortified with calcium, and pumpkin seeds are vegan sources of iron.
- **Consideration:** To improve iron absorption, combine meals high in iron with foods high in vitamin C, such as citrus fruits, bell peppers, and strawberries. Think about including foods high in iron during meals and snacks all throughout the day.

Calcium

-**Importance:** The growth of a fetus's teeth and bones, as well as the health of a mother's bones, depend on calcium.

- **Food Sources:** Fortified plant milks (soy, almond, and oat), tofu set with calcium sulfate, fortified orange juice, broccoli, bok choy, kale, collard greens, sesame seeds, and tahini are vegan sources of calcium.

- **Consideration:** Try to get enough calcium from a mix of naturally high-calcium plant sources and fortified meals. Incorporate foods high in calcium into your meals and snacks to aid with absorption.

Omega-3 Fatty Acids

- **Importance:** DHA (docosahexaenoic acid), in particular, is essential for the development of the fetus's brain and eyes.
- **Food Sources:** Algae oil, walnuts, flaxseeds, chia seeds, hemp seeds, and fortified foods (such plant-based milk and yogurt) are vegan sources of omega-3 fatty acids.
- **Considerations:** To guarantee sufficient intake, particularly if dietary sources are restricted, think about including omega-3-rich foods in regular meals or thinking about taking supplements based on algae for DHA.

Vitamin B12

- **Importance:** B12 is necessary for the development of the nervous system and the prevention of congenital abnormalities.

- **Food Sources:** Fortified foods (such nutritional yeast, fortified plant milks, morning cereals, and meat alternatives) and vitamin B12 supplements are vegan sources of vitamin B12.

- **Consideration:** Pregnant vegans should make sure they are getting enough vitamin B12 via fortified meals or supplements, since the vitamin is mostly found in animal sources. This will help avoid deficiency.

Folate

- **Importance:** Folate, or vitamin B9, is essential for shielding the developing embryo against neural tube abnormalities.

- **Food Sources:** Leafy greens (kale, spinach), lentils, beans, avocado, broccoli, citrus fruits, and fortified grains are vegan sources of folate.

- **Consideration:** Try to eat a diversified diet full of foods high in folate, and if your doctor advises it, you should also think about taking a folic acid supplement.

Zinc

- **Importance:** Zinc is necessary for both immunological system performance and fetal growth and development.
- **Food Sources:** Legumes, nuts, seeds, whole grains, tofu, tempeh, and fortified cereals are vegan sources of zinc.
- **Consideration:** Make sure you consume enough foods high in zinc throughout your pregnancy, and if possible, combine plant-based sources of zinc with sources of vitamin C to improve absorption.

Vitamin D

- **Importance:** Vitamin D is required for the health of your bones and the absorption of calcium.

- **Food Sources:** Fortified plant milks, fortified orange juice, fortified cereals, sun-exposed mushrooms, and vitamin D supplements are among the vegan sources of vitamin D.

- **Consideration:** Since hardly many foods are naturally high in vitamin D, think about including foods that have been fortified with the vitamin and talking to your doctor about supplements, especially if you don't get much sunshine.

- **Supplementation**

To satisfy your unique dietary demands during pregnancy, talk to your doctor about whether prenatal supplements are essential. as well as the right supplement amounts according to certain requirements and situations.
- To guarantee the best possible health results for both mother and child, pregnant vegans may need to supplement with specific nutrients, such as vitamin B12, vitamin D, iron, and omega-3 fatty acids.

Meal Planning for a Healthy Vegan Pregnancy

To promote the health of both the mother and the fetus and to fulfill the increased nutritional demands during pregnancy, meal planning is essential. In order to provide the best possible nutrition, vegan expectant women must carefully examine meals high in nutrients. Here's how to prepare meals for a healthy vegan pregnancy, step-by-step:

1. Evaluate Nutritional Needs: - Speak with a medical professional or registered dietitian to find out what nutrients you specifically need depending on your age, weight, amount of exercise, and any underlying medical concerns.

2. Prepare Balanced Meals and Snacks: - To get a broad range of nutrients, aim for a selection of plant-based meals in each meal.

- Add protein-rich foods like quinoa, almonds, seeds, tempeh, beans, lentils, tofu, and edamame.

- For fiber, energy, and vital nutrients, include whole grains such as brown rice, quinoa, oats, barley, whole wheat pasta, and whole grain bread.

- Incorporate an abundance of colorful fruits and vegetables to provide fiber, vitamins, minerals, and antioxidants.

- Incorporate healthy fats for hormone synthesis and brain development from foods like avocados, nuts, seeds, olives, and plant-based oils.

- To keep your energy levels consistent throughout the day, divide your daily food consumption into three major meals (breakfast, lunch, and supper) and two to three snacks.

- Prepare nutrient-dense, filling snacks, including a small handful of nuts and seeds, whole grain crackers with hummus, fresh fruit with nut butter, or veggie sticks with guacamole.

3. Remain Hydrated: Throughout the day, sip on plenty of water to maintain proper circulation, digestion, and nutritional absorption.

   - In addition to offering diversity to your drinks, herbal teas, coconut water, and homemade fruit-infused water may help you stay hydrated.

4. Be Flexible and Pay Attention to Your Body: - Cravings and aversions throughout pregnancy are typical, so be adaptable with your diet plan and pay attention to your body's cues.

   - Incorporate a range of tastes and meals to satiate appetites and fulfill dietary requirements.

   - If you suffer from nausea or other digestive issues, prioritize foods that are simple to digest and smaller, more frequent meals.

Chapter 2

Managing Blood Sugar Levels: Tips and Tricks for Diabetic-Friendly Eating

Choose Low Glycemic Index (GI) Foods:
- Selecting foods with a low glycemic index can help prevent spikes in blood sugar levels. Low GI foods include non-starchy vegetables (such as leafy greens, broccoli, cauliflower), legumes (beans, lentils), whole grains (quinoa, barley, oats), and most fruits (such as berries, apples, citrus fruits).

Balance Carbohydrates with Protein and Healthy Fats:
- Pairing carbohydrates with protein and healthy fats can slow down the absorption of glucose into the bloodstream, preventing rapid spikes in blood sugar levels. For example, pair whole grain toast with

avocado and tofu, or have a small serving of fruit with nuts or seeds.

Monitor Portion Sizes:

- Pay attention to portion sizes to avoid overconsumption of carbohydrates, which can lead to elevated blood sugar levels. Use measuring cups, food scales, or visual cues to estimate appropriate portion sizes, especially for carbohydrate-rich foods like grains, fruits, and starchy vegetables.

Eat Regular Meals and Snacks:

- Consuming regular meals and snacks throughout the day can help stabilize blood sugar levels and prevent large fluctuations. Aim to eat every 3-4 hours to maintain consistent energy levels and avoid prolonged periods of hunger, which can lead to overeating or unhealthy food choices.

Focus on Fiber-Rich Foods:

   - Fiber slows down the digestion and absorption of carbohydrates, resulting in more stable blood sugar levels. Include plenty of fiber-rich foods in your diet, such as vegetables, fruits, legumes, whole grains, nuts, and seeds. Aim for a variety of soluble and insoluble fiber sources for optimal health benefits.

Limit Added Sugars and Refined Carbohydrates:

   - Minimize the intake of foods and beverages high in added sugars and refined carbohydrates, such as sugary drinks, desserts, candies, pastries, and white bread. These foods can cause rapid spikes in blood sugar levels and contribute to insulin resistance over time.

Stay Hydrated with Water:

   - Drinking an adequate amount of water throughout the day is essential for hydration and can help regulate blood sugar levels.

Opt for water as your primary beverage choice and limit the consumption of sugary drinks, which can contribute to blood sugar spikes.

Monitor Blood Sugar Levels Regularly:
- Keep track of your blood sugar levels as directed by your healthcare provider using a blood glucose monitor. Regular monitoring can help you understand how different foods and lifestyle factors affect your blood sugar levels and allow for timely adjustments to your diet and medication regimen.

Work with a Registered Dietitian or Certified Diabetes Educator:
- Collaborate with a healthcare professional, such as a registered dietitian or certified diabetes educator, to develop a personalized meal plan and learn strategies for managing blood sugar levels effectively during pregnancy. They can provide guidance on carbohydrate counting, meal

timing, and food choices tailored to your individual needs and preferences.

Managing Morning Sickness and Other Pregnancy Challenges with Vegan Foods

Choose Simple, Easily Digestible Foods:
- Choose mild, easily digestible vegan meals that are less likely to make you sick to your stomach. Simple crackers, bread, rice, applesauce, bananas, and broth-based soups are a few examples.

Add Ginger:
- Studies have shown that ginger may help reduce nausea and vomiting in pregnant women. To help ease upset stomachs, consider adding fresh ginger to meals, drinks, and smoothies. You may also try ginger pills or ginger sweets.

Remain Hydrated:

- Throughout the day, consume clear drinks to remain hydrated and avoid dehydration, which may make nausea worse. Soothsaying drinks include diluted fruit juices, herbal teas, coconut water, and ginger ale (ideally non-alcoholic).

Consume Small, Regular Meals:

- Small, frequent snacks or mini-meals should be consumed throughout the day in place of larger meals to maintain stable blood sugar levels and avoid nausea. Give special attention to nutrient-dense vegan meals including smoothies, whole grain crackers, nuts, and seeds, as well as dried fruits.

Steer away from Strong Odors and Trigger Foods:

- Foods with strong aromas or excessive spice should be avoided as they may intensify nausea. Choose mild, neutral-flavored vegan choices in place of morning sickness trigger foods by identifying and avoiding them.

Try Various Plant-Based Protein Sources:
- Try switching to more readily digested plant-based protein sources if you have trouble tolerating meals high in protein due to morning sickness. Think about legumes (like chickpeas and lentils), tofu, tempeh, or protein-packed smoothies made with silken tofu or vegan protein powder.

Pay Attention to the Nutrients You Eat:
-   In spite of nausea and food allergies, make an effort to get enough nutrients by consuming nutrient-dense vegan meals whenever you can. To make sure that your pregnant body gets all the vital nutrients it needs, concentrate on eating a wide range of fruits, vegetables, whole grains, nuts, seeds, and plant-based proteins.

Take Supplements if Needed:

- Speak with a healthcare professional about the possibility of taking prenatal vitamins or particular nutrients like vitamin B6, vitamin B12, or iron to address potential deficiencies if morning sickness has a significant impact on food intake and nutrient absorption.

Seek Support and Rest:

- To deal with the difficulties of morning sickness and other pregnancy symptoms, prioritize self-care and ask for help from family, friends, and medical professionals. Remind yourself to take breaks, pay attention to your body's cues, and don't be afraid to seek assistance when you need it.

Chapter 3

Recipes for Pregnancy

Breakfast Recipes

1. Tofu and Vegetable Scramble:

Ingredients:

- 1 block (14 oz) firm tofu, drained and crumbled
- 1 tablespoon olive oil
- ½ onion, diced
- 1 bell pepper, diced
- 1 cup mushrooms, sliced
- 2 cups spinach leaves
- 2 cloves garlic, minced
- ½ teaspoon turmeric powder
- Salt and pepper to taste
- Optional: nutritional yeast for added flavor

Instructions:

- In a large pan set over medium heat, warm the olive oil. Saute the bell peppers and onions for three to four minutes, or until they are tender.
- Add the mushrooms and garlic to the skillet and simmer for 2 to 3 minutes, or until the mushrooms are soft.
- Stir well to blend the turmeric and crumbled tofu in the skillet. Cook for a further five to six minutes, or until the tofu is well cooked and beginning to become golden.
- Add the spinach leaves and simmer for one to two minutes, or until wilted. If preferred, add nutritional yeast and salt and pepper for seasoning.
- If preferred, top hot dish with fresh herbs.

2. Chickpea Flour Pancakes with Berries:

Ingredients:

- 1 cup chickpea flour
- 1 tablespoon ground flaxseed
- 1 tablespoon maple syrup or sweetener of choice
- 1 teaspoon baking powder
- ½ teaspoon cinnamon
- Pinch of salt
- 1 cup almond milk
- ½ cup mixed berries (blueberries, raspberries, strawberries)

Instructions:

- Mix the chickpea flour, ground flaxseed, maple syrup, baking powder, cinnamon, and salt in a large mixing dish.
- Add almond milk gradually while stirring to create a smooth batter. To thicken, let the batter sit for five to ten minutes.

- Turn up the heat to medium on a nonstick skillet or griddle. For each pancake, add ¼ cup of batter to the skillet.
- Cook the pancake for one to two more minutes, or until golden brown, after flipping it once bubbles start to appear on the top.
- Proceed with the leftover batter. Warm pancakes should be served with mixed berries and more maple syrup, if preferred.

3. Chia Seed Pudding with Almond Milk:

Ingredients:

- ¼ cup chia seeds
- 1 cup almond milk
- 1 tablespoon maple syrup or sweetener of choice
- ½ teaspoon vanilla extract
- Optional toppings: sliced almonds, fresh berries, shredded coconut

Instructions:

- Chia seeds, almond milk, maple syrup, and vanilla extract should all be combined in a mixing dish. Mix well to blend.
- To enable the chia seeds to soak up the liquid and thicken, cover the bowl and place it in the refrigerator for at least two hours, or better yet, overnight.
- To guarantee a uniform consistency, give the pudding a stir before serving. You may modify the thickness by adding additional almond milk if required.
- Spoon the chia seed pudding into each serving dish, then garnish with shredded coconut, fresh berries, and almond slices. Present cold.

4. Tempeh Bacon and Avocado Toast:

Ingredients:

- 4 slices whole grain bread, toasted
- 1 avocado, sliced
- 1 package tempeh (8 oz), thinly sliced
- 1 tablespoon soy sauce or tamari
- 1 tablespoon maple syrup
- ½ teaspoon smoked paprika
- ¼ teaspoon garlic powder
- Salt and pepper to taste
- Optional toppings: sliced tomato, microgreens

Instructions:

- To create the marinade, mix together soy sauce, maple syrup, garlic powder, smoked paprika, salt, and pepper in a small bowl.
- Transfer the marinade-covered tempeh slices to a shallow dish, making sure that every piece is equally covered. Give it at least fifteen minutes to marinate.

- Turn on a medium heat source for a nonstick skillet. Place the marinated tempeh slices in the pan and cook for 3–4 minutes on each side, or until crispy and golden brown.
- Spread sliced avocado on pieces of toasted bread to construct the avocado toast. Add cooked tempeh bacon on the top of each piece.
- If preferred, garnish with sliced tomato and microgreens. Serve right away.

5. Vegan Protein Smoothie with Spinach and Banana:

Ingredients:

- 1 ripe banana
- 1 cup fresh spinach leaves
- 1 tablespoon almond butter or peanut butter
- 1 scoop vegan protein powder (flavor of your choice)

- 1 cup unsweetened almond milk
- Ice cubes (optional)

Instructions:

- Blend together the banana, almond butter, vegan protein powder, spinach leaves, and almond milk using a blender.
- Process on high speed until creamy and smooth. If you would want your smoothie cooler, add ice cubes.
- Assess sweetness and make necessary adjustments.

6. Quinoa Breakfast Bowl with Almonds and Fruit:

Ingredients:

- ½ cup quinoa
- 1 cup almond milk (or any plant-based milk)
- ¼ teaspoon ground cinnamon

- ¼ teaspoon vanilla extract
- 1 tablespoon maple syrup (optional)
- 2 tablespoons sliced almonds
- ½ cup mixed berries (such as strawberries, blueberries, raspberries)
- Fresh mint leaves for garnish (optional)

Instructions:

- Rinse the quinoa with a fine-mesh strainer under cold water.
- Place the rinsed quinoa, almond milk, vanilla extract, and cinnamon in a small saucepan.
- After bringing the mixture to a boil, lower the heat to a simmer, cover it, and cook the quinoa for 15 to 20 minutes, or until it is tender and the liquid has been absorbed.
- After cooking, use a fork to fluff the quinoa and, if desired, toss in the maple syrup.
- Spoon cooked quinoa into dishes for dishing. Place mixed berries and sliced almonds on top of each bowl.

- If preferred, garnish with fresh mint leaves and serve warm.

7. Lentil Breakfast Patties with Roasted Vegetables:

Ingredients:

- 1 cup cooked lentils
- ½ cup breadcrumbs (gluten-free if needed)
- 1 flax egg (1 tablespoon ground flaxseed + 3 tablespoons water)
- ¼ cup finely chopped onion
- 1 garlic clove, minced
- ½ teaspoon ground cumin
- ½ teaspoon paprika
- Salt and pepper to taste
- 2 tablespoons olive oil
- Roasted vegetables of your choice (such as bell peppers, zucchini, cherry tomatoes)

Instructions:

- Turn the oven on to 375°F, or 190°C. Use parchment paper to line a baking sheet.
- Put the cooked lentils, breadcrumbs, flax egg, minced garlic, diced onion, ground cumin, paprika, salt, and pepper in a big mixing bowl. Blend until well blended.
- Using the lentil mixture, form patties and transfer to the baking sheet that has been preheated.
- Lightly coat both sides of the patties with olive oil.
- Bake for 20 to 25 minutes in a preheated oven, rotating the patties halfway through, or until they are crispy and golden brown.
- Present the lentil patties with roasted veggies.

8. Almond Butter Banana Oatmeal:

Ingredients:

- ½ cup rolled oats
- 1 cup water or almond milk
- 1 ripe banana, mashed
- 2 tablespoons almond butter
- 1 tablespoon maple syrup or sweetener of choice (optional)
- Pinch of cinnamon
- Sliced almonds for garnish (optional)

Instructions:

- Rollin oats and water or almond milk should be combined in a small pot. After bringing to a boil, lower the heat to a simmer and cook the oats for five to seven minutes, stirring now and again, until they are soft and cooked.
- Add the almond butter, cinnamon, maple syrup (if using), and mashed banana and stir until thoroughly blended.

- Cook for a further one to two minutes, or until well cooked.
- Take the oatmeal off of the stove and place it in serving dishes.
- If preferred, garnish with chopped almonds and serve warm.

9. Vegan Breakfast Tacos with Black Beans and Salsa:

Ingredients:

- 4 small corn tortillas
- 1 cup cooked black beans
- 1 ripe avocado, sliced
- Salsa of your choice
- Fresh cilantro leaves for garnish (optional)
- Lime wedges for serving

Instructions:

- In a dry pan, cook the corn tortillas for one to two minutes on each side, or until they are well cooked and softened.
- Stuff each tortilla with salsa, chopped avocado, and cooked black beans.
- Serve with lime wedges on the side and garnish with fresh cilantro leaves, if preferred.

10. Oat Bran Porridge with Flaxseed and Berries:

Ingredients:

- ½ cup oat bran
- 1 cup water or plant-based milk
- 1 tablespoon ground flaxseed
- 1 tablespoon maple syrup or sweetener of choice
- ½ cup mixed berries (such as strawberries, blueberries, raspberries)

- 1 tablespoon chopped nuts or seeds for garnish (optional)

Instructions:

- Heat the plant-based milk or water in a small pot until it boils.
- Turn down the heat and stir in the oat bran. Cook, stirring periodically, until the porridge thickens, 3 to 5 minutes.
- Ensure that the ground flaxseed and maple syrup are well mixed together.
- Take the oat bran porridge from the stove and place it in serving dishes.
- As a garnish, add chopped nuts or seeds and a mixture of berries on top.
- Present warm.

Lunch Recipes

1. Lentil Soup with Vegetables:

Ingredients:

- 1 cup dried green lentils
- 4 cups vegetable broth
- 1 onion, diced
- 2 carrots, diced
- 2 celery stalks, diced
- 2 cloves garlic, minced
- 1 teaspoon ground cumin
- 1 teaspoon ground turmeric
- ½ teaspoon smoked paprika
- Salt and pepper to taste
- 2 cups chopped spinach or kale
- Juice of 1 lemon
- Fresh parsley for garnish (optional)

Instructions:

- After rinsing with cold water, drain the lentils.
- Heat some olive oil in a big saucepan over medium heat. Cook the chopped onion, carrots, and celery for 5 to 7 minutes, or until they are tender.
- Cook the smoked paprika, cumin, turmeric, and minced garlic for a further one to two minutes, or until aromatic.
- Add the lentils and pour in the vegetable broth. After bringing the soup to a boil, lower the heat to a simmer, cover it, and let it cook for 20 to 25 minutes, or until the lentils are soft.
- Add the chopped kale or spinach and simmer, stirring, until the greens wilt, about 5 more minutes.
- Turn off the heat and whisk in the lemon juice. To taste, add salt and pepper for seasoning.
- If desired, top the hot dish with fresh parsley.

2. Chickpea Salad with Lemon Tahini Dressing:

Ingredients:

- 1 can (15 oz) chickpeas, drained and rinsed
- 1 cucumber, diced
- 1 red bell pepper, diced
- ¼ cup diced red onion
- ¼ cup chopped fresh parsley
- Juice of 1 lemon
- 2 tablespoons tahini
- 1 tablespoon olive oil
- 1 clove garlic, minced
- Salt and pepper to taste

Instructions:

- Chickpeas, diced onion, diced bell pepper, diced cucumber, and chopped fresh parsley should all be combined in a big mixing dish.
- To create the dressing, combine the olive oil, tahini, lemon juice, chopped garlic, salt, and pepper in a small bowl.

- Drizzle the chickpea salad with the dressing and mix well.
- Taste and, if necessary, adjust seasoning.
- You may serve chilled or at room temperature.

3. Tofu Stir-Fry with Broccoli and Bell Peppers:

Ingredients:

- 1 block (14 oz) extra-firm tofu, pressed and cubed
- 2 tablespoons soy sauce or tamari
- 1 tablespoon sesame oil
- 1 tablespoon cornstarch
- 1 tablespoon olive oil
- 2 cups broccoli florets
- 1 red bell pepper, sliced
- 1 yellow bell pepper, sliced
- 2 cloves garlic, minced
- 1 tablespoon grated ginger
- Cooked rice or quinoa for serving

- Sesame seeds for garnish (optional)
- Green onions for garnish (optional)

Instructions:

- To create the marinade, combine the cornstarch, sesame oil, and soy sauce in a small bowl.
- Heat the olive oil in a big pan or wok over medium-high heat. Add the cubed tofu and heat for 5 to 7 minutes, or until golden brown on both sides. After taking the tofu out of the pan, put it aside.
- Place the cut bell peppers and broccoli florets in the same pan. Simmer for 4–5 minutes, or until crisp-tender.
- Cook the grated ginger and minced garlic in the pan for a further one to two minutes, or until fragrant.
- Transfer the cooked tofu back to the pan and cover the tofu and veggies with the marinade. To uniformly coat everything, give it a good stir.

- Simmer for a further two to three minutes, or until the sauce is thicker.
- Top the heated tofu stir-fry with quinoa or cooked rice.
- If preferred, garnish with sliced green onions and sesame seeds.

4. Quinoa Salad with Black Beans and Corn:

Ingredients:

- 1 cup quinoa
- 2 cups water or vegetable broth
- 1 can (15 oz) black beans, drained and rinsed
- 1 cup cooked corn kernels (fresh, frozen, or canned)
- 1 red bell pepper, diced
- ¼ cup chopped fresh cilantro
- Juice of 1 lime
- 2 tablespoons olive oil
- Salt and pepper to taste

- Avocado slices for garnish (optional)

Instructions:

- After rinsing with cold water, drain the quinoa.
- Put the quinoa and the vegetable broth or water in a medium pot. After bringing to a boil, lower the heat to a simmer, cover, and cook the quinoa for 15 to 20 minutes, or until it is tender and the liquid has been absorbed.
- Use a fork to fluff the quinoa before adding it to a big mixing bowl.
- Combine the quinoa with the black beans, cooked corn kernels, diced red bell pepper, and fresh cilantro that has been chopped.
- To create the dressing, combine the lime juice, olive oil, salt, and pepper in a small bowl.
- Drizzle the quinoa salad with the dressing and toss to fully incorporate.
- Taste and, if necessary, adjust seasoning.

- You may serve it cold or at room temperature and top it with avocado slices if you'd like.

5. Vegan Chili with Kidney Beans and Sweet Potatoes:

Ingredients:

- 1 tablespoon olive oil
- 1 onion, diced
- 2 cloves garlic, minced
- 1 sweet potato, peeled and diced
- 1 red bell pepper, diced
- 1 can (15 oz) diced tomatoes
- 1 can (15 oz) kidney beans, drained and rinsed
- 2 cups vegetable broth
- 1 tablespoon chili powder
- 1 teaspoon ground cumin
- 1 teaspoon smoked paprika
- Salt and pepper to taste
- Fresh cilantro for garnish (optional)

- Avocado slices for serving (optional)

Instructions:

- Heat the olive oil in a big saucepan over medium heat. Add the chopped onion and garlic, and simmer for approximately 5 minutes, or until softened.
- Cook the red bell pepper and chopped sweet potato in the saucepan for a further five minutes, or until the potatoes start to soften.
- Add the smoked paprika, cumin, chili powder, chopped tomatoes, kidney beans, vegetable broth, salt, and pepper.
- After bringing the chili to a boil, lower the heat to a simmer and cook, stirring from time to time, until the flavors have blended and the sweet potatoes are soft, 20 to 25 minutes.
- Taste and, if necessary, adjust seasoning.
- Present the vegan chili hot, topped with avocado slices and fresh cilantro, if preferred.

6. Tempeh Lettuce Wraps with Avocado:

Ingredients:

- 1 package (8 oz) tempeh, crumbled
- 2 tablespoons soy sauce or tamari
- 1 tablespoon sesame oil
- 1 tablespoon rice vinegar
- 1 tablespoon maple syrup
- 1 teaspoon grated ginger
- 1 clove garlic, minced
- ¼ teaspoon red pepper flakes (optional)
- 1 avocado, sliced
- Lettuce leaves for wrapping (such as butter lettuce or romaine)
- Sliced cucumber, shredded carrots, chopped green onions for topping (optional)

Instructions:

- Combine the soy sauce, sesame oil, rice vinegar, maple syrup, chopped garlic, grated ginger, and red pepper flakes (if using) in a small bowl.
- Turn the heat down to medium in a nonstick skillet. Cover with the marinade and add the crushed tempeh.
- Cook the tempeh for five to seven minutes, stirring now and again, until it's well cooked and marinated.
- Take the skillet off of the burner and let the tempeh cool a little.
- Spoon a little of the tempeh mixture over each lettuce leaf to make the lettuce wraps.
- If preferred, garnish with sliced cucumber, sliced avocado, shredded carrots, and chopped green onions.
- If necessary, use toothpicks to bind the lettuce leaves as you roll them up.
- Present the lettuce wraps with tempeh right away.

7. Cauliflower Rice Bowl with Tofu and Mixed Vegetables:

Ingredients:

- 1 block (14 oz) extra-firm tofu, pressed and cubed
- 1 tablespoon soy sauce or tamari
- 1 tablespoon sesame oil
- 1 tablespoon olive oil
- 1 head cauliflower, grated or processed into rice
- 2 cups mixed vegetables (such as bell peppers, broccoli, carrots, snap peas)
- 2 cloves garlic, minced
- 1 tablespoon grated ginger
- Cooked brown rice or quinoa for serving
- Sesame seeds and chopped green onions for garnish (optional)

Instructions:

- Put the cubed tofu, sesame oil, and soy sauce in a small bowl. Give it 10 to 15 minutes to marinate.
- In a large skillet or wok, heat the olive oil over medium heat. After adding the marinated tofu cubes, heat for 5 to 7 minutes, or until golden brown on both sides. Take out the tofu and put it aside in a skillet.
- Place the mixed veggies and shredded cauliflower rice in the same skillet. Cook the veggies for 5 to 7 minutes, or until they are crisp-tender.
- Add the grated ginger and minced garlic, and simmer for a further one to two minutes, or until fragrant.
- Add the cooked tofu back to the pan and stir everything until it is well heated.
- Top cooked quinoa or brown rice with the cauliflower rice and tofu combination.
- If preferred, garnish with chopped green onions and sesame seeds.

8. Mediterranean Lentil Salad with Spinach and Olives:

Ingredients:

- 1 cup green lentils, cooked and drained
- 2 cups baby spinach leaves
- ½ cup cherry tomatoes, halved
- ¼ cup sliced Kalamata olives
- ¼ cup diced red onion
- 2 tablespoons chopped fresh parsley
- 2 tablespoons extra virgin olive oil
- 1 tablespoon red wine vinegar
- 1 teaspoon Dijon mustard
- Salt and pepper to taste
- Crumbled vegan feta cheese for topping (optional)

Instructions:

- Cooked lentils, baby spinach leaves, cherry tomatoes, diced red onion, sliced Kalamata olives, and chopped fresh parsley should all be combined in a large mixing dish.

- To create the dressing, combine the extra virgin olive oil, red wine vinegar, Dijon mustard, salt, and pepper in a small bowl.
- Drizzle the lentil salad with the dressing and mix well.
- Taste and, if necessary, adjust seasoning.
- You may serve the chilled or room temperature Mediterranean lentil salad with crumbled vegan feta cheese on top if you'd like.

9. Vegan Buddha Bowl with Roasted Vegetables and Hummus:

Ingredients:

- 1 cup quinoa, rinsed
- 2 cups water or vegetable broth
- 1 large sweet potato, peeled and diced
- 2 cups cauliflower florets
- 1 red bell pepper, sliced
- 1 tablespoon olive oil
- Salt and pepper, to taste

- 2 cups mixed greens or spinach
- 1 cup cherry tomatoes, halved
- ½ cup cucumber, sliced
- ¼ cup sliced red onion
- ¼ cup hummus
- 2 tablespoons tahini
- Juice of 1 lemon
- 2 tablespoons chopped fresh parsley or cilantro (optional)

Instructions:

- Set oven temperature to 400°F, or 200°C.
- Put the quinoa and the vegetable broth or water in a saucepan. After bringing to a boil, lower the heat to a simmer, cover, and cook the quinoa for 15 to 20 minutes, or until it is tender and the liquid has been absorbed.
- Arrange the sliced red bell pepper, chopped sweet potato, and cauliflower florets on a baking pan and cook the quinoa. Season with salt and pepper and drizzle with olive oil. Roast the veggies for 20 to 25

minutes in a preheated oven, or until they are soft and have a light brown hue.

- In a separate bowl, mix together the hummus, tahini, and lemon juice to create the dressing.

- Distribute the cooked quinoa among serving dishes to construct the Buddha bowls. Add roasted veggies, red onion, cucumber, cherry tomatoes, and mixed greens on top.

- Cover the bowls with a drizzle of hummus and tahini dressing.

- If preferred, garnish with finely chopped fresh cilantro or parsley.

- Present the heated Buddha bowls and enjoy them!

10. Black Bean Tacos with Mango Salsa:

Ingredients:

For the black bean filling:
- 1 can (15 oz) black beans, drained and rinsed
- 1 tablespoon olive oil
- 1 small onion, diced
- 2 cloves garlic, minced
- 1 teaspoon ground cumin
- 1 teaspoon chili powder
- Salt and pepper, to taste
- ¼ cup water

For the mango salsa:
- 1 ripe mango, peeled and diced
- ½ red onion, finely chopped
- ¼ cup chopped fresh cilantro
- Juice of 1 lime
- Salt and pepper, to taste

For serving:
- 8 small corn or flour tortillas
- Optional toppings: shredded lettuce, diced avocado, sliced jalapenos, vegan sour cream, lime wedges

Instructions:

- Heat the olive oil in a pan over medium heat. Add the chopped onion and simmer for 3–4 minutes, or until transparent. Sauté the minced garlic for a further minute.
- Fill the pan with black beans, chili powder, ground cumin, salt, and pepper. Mix everything together.
- After adding the water, boil the mixture in the skillet for five to seven minutes, or until it is well cooked and has thickened somewhat. If desired, use the back of a spoon to mash some of the beans for a thicker consistency.
- To create the mango salsa, place the diced mango, red onion, cilantro, lime juice, salt, and pepper in a bowl. Mix well to blend.

- Reheat tortillas in the microwave or on a dry pan as directed on the box.
- Spoon each tortilla with black bean filling to create the tacos. Add mango salsa and any preferred toppings on top.
- Serve right away and savor your delicious mango salsa with black bean tacos!

Dinner Recipes

1. Lentil Shepherd's Pie:

Ingredients:

- 1 cup dry green or brown lentils
- 2 cups vegetable broth
- 2 tablespoons olive oil
- 1 onion, diced
- 2 carrots, diced
- 2 stalks celery, diced
- 2 cloves garlic, minced
- 1 teaspoon dried thyme
- 1 teaspoon dried rosemary
- Salt and pepper to taste
- 4 cups mashed potatoes (made from about 4 large potatoes)
- 1 tablespoon vegan butter (optional)
- Fresh parsley for garnish (optional)

Instructions:

- Turn the oven on to 375°F, or 190°C.
- Drain and rinse the lentils in cold water.
- Place the lentils and vegetable broth in a saucepan. After bringing to a boil, simmer the lentils for 20 to 25 minutes, covered, or until they are soft and the liquid has been absorbed.
- Heat the olive oil in a big pan over medium heat. Add the minced garlic, chopped onion, carrots, and celery. Simmer the veggies for five to seven minutes, or until they are tender.
- Add the salt, pepper, dried thyme, and dry rosemary to the cooked lentils. Remove from heat and cook for a further two to three minutes.
- Transfer and level out the lentil mixture in a baking dish.
- Using a spatula, evenly distribute the mashed potatoes over the lentil mixture.

- Bake for 25 to 30 minutes in a preheated oven, or until the tops of the mashed potatoes are golden brown.
- Take it out of the oven and let it cool down a few minutes before serving.
- If wanted, garnish with fresh parsley and serve hot.

2. Baked Tofu with Steamed Broccoli:

Ingredients:

- 1 block (14 oz) extra-firm tofu, pressed and sliced into cubes
- 2 tablespoons soy sauce or tamari
- 1 tablespoon olive oil
- 1 teaspoon garlic powder
- 1 teaspoon onion powder
- ½ teaspoon smoked paprika
- Salt and pepper to taste
- 4 cups broccoli florets

Instructions:

- Set oven temperature to 400°F, or 200°C. Use parchment paper to line a baking sheet.
- Combine soy sauce, olive oil, smoked paprika, onion and garlic powders, salt, and pepper in a bowl.
- Place the tofu cubes in the basin and toss them slightly to evenly distribute the marinade.
- Evenly distribute the marinated tofu cubes on the baking sheet that has been ready.
- Bake for 25 to 30 minutes in a preheated oven, rotating the tofu halfway through, or until it becomes crispy and golden brown.
- Steam the broccoli florets for five to seven minutes, or until they are soft, while the tofu bakes.
- Present the cooked tofu with steaming broccoli.

3. Chickpea and Vegetable Stir-Fry:

Ingredients:

- 1 tablespoon sesame oil
- 1 onion, sliced
- 2 cloves garlic, minced
- 1 bell pepper, sliced
- 1 cup sliced mushrooms
- 1 cup snap peas, trimmed
- 1 can (15 oz) chickpeas, drained and rinsed
- 2 tablespoons soy sauce or tamari
- 1 tablespoon rice vinegar
- 1 tablespoon maple syrup or sweetener of choice
- Cooked rice or quinoa for serving
- Sesame seeds and sliced green onions for garnish (optional)

Instructions:

- In a big skillet or wok, warm up the sesame oil over medium heat.
- Fill the pan with minced garlic and chopped onion. Simmer for three to four minutes, or until the onion is tender.
- Fill the pan with the sliced bell pepper, snap peas, and mushrooms. Stir-fry the veggies for five to seven minutes, or until they are crisp-tender.
- Add the rinsed and drained chickpeas and stir.
- Combine the soy sauce, rice vinegar, and maple syrup in a small basin. Over the veggies and chickpeas in the pan, pour the sauce.
- Cook for a further two to three minutes, stirring now and again, until the sauce has thickened and the food is well cooked.
- Top cooked rice or quinoa with the stir-fried veggies and chickpeas.
- If preferred, garnish with sliced green onions and sesame seeds.

4. Stuffed Bell Peppers with Quinoa and Black Beans:

Ingredients:

- 4 bell peppers, any color
- 1 cup cooked quinoa
- 1 can (15 oz) black beans, drained and rinsed
- 1 cup corn kernels (fresh, frozen, or canned)
- 1 cup diced tomatoes
- ½ cup diced red onion
- 2 cloves garlic, minced
- 1 teaspoon ground cumin
- 1 teaspoon chili powder
- Salt and pepper to taste
- ½ cup shredded vegan cheese (optional)
- Fresh cilantro for garnish (optional)

Instructions:

- Turn the oven on to 375°F, or 190°C. Coat a baking dish with oil.
- Slice off the bell peppers' tops, then take out the seeds and membranes.
- Put cooked quinoa, black beans, corn kernels, chopped tomatoes, chopped red onion, minced garlic, ground cumin, chili powder, salt, and pepper in a big mixing bowl.
- Fill the hollowed-out bell peppers with the quinoa and black bean mixture.
- Transfer the filled bell peppers to the baking dish that has been ready.
- Top the filled bell peppers with shredded vegan cheese, if using.
- Bake the baking dish for 25 to 30 minutes in a preheated oven covered with aluminum foil.
- Take off the foil and bake for a further five to ten minutes, or until the mixture is well cooked and the bell peppers are soft.

- If preferred, garnish with fresh cilantro and serve hot.

5. Vegan Lentil Loaf with Mashed Cauliflower:

Ingredients:

For the lentil loaf:
- 1 cup dry green or brown lentils
- 2 cups vegetable broth
- 1 tablespoon olive oil
- 1 onion, diced
- 2 cloves garlic, minced
- 1 carrot, grated
- 1 celery stalk, diced
- 1 tablespoon tomato paste
- 1 tablespoon soy sauce or tamari
- 1 teaspoon dried thyme
- 1 teaspoon dried rosemary
- ½ teaspoon smoked paprika
- Salt and pepper to taste
- ½ cup rolled oats

- ¼ cup ground flaxseed
- ¼ cup chopped fresh parsley

For the mashed cauliflower:
- 1 head cauliflower, cut into florets
- 2 cloves garlic, minced
- 2 tablespoons vegan butter
- Salt and pepper to taste

Instructions:

- Turn the oven on to 375°F, or 190°C. Apply grease to a loaf pan.
- Drain and rinse the lentils in cold water.
- Place the lentils and vegetable broth in a saucepan. After bringing to a boil, simmer the lentils for 20 to 25 minutes, covered, or until they are soft and the liquid has been absorbed.
- Heat the olive oil in a pan over medium heat. Add the chopped celery, grated carrot, minced garlic, and onion. Cook for five to seven minutes, or until tender.

- Add the smoked paprika, tomato paste, soy sauce, dried thyme, and dried rosemary. Simmer for a further two to three minutes.
- Place the cooked lentils, cooked vegetable combination, rolled oats, ground flaxseed, and parsley in a large mixing dish. Blend until well blended.
- Pour the lentil mixture into the loaf pan that has been preheated and firmly push it down.
- Bake for 40 to 45 minutes, or until the top of the lentil loaf is golden brown and hard, in a preheated oven.
- Steam the cauliflower florets for ten to fifteen minutes, or until they are soft, while the lentil loaf is baking.
- Place the cooked cauliflower in a basin and mash it smooth with vegan butter, chopped garlic, salt, and pepper.
- Present portions of lentil loaf accompanied by a substantial portion of creamy cauliflower on the side.

6. Eggplant Lasagna with Tofu Ricotta:

Ingredients:

For the tofu ricotta:
- 1 block (14 oz) extra-firm tofu, drained
- 2 tablespoons nutritional yeast
- 1 tablespoon lemon juice
- 1 teaspoon dried basil
- 1 teaspoon dried oregano
- Salt and pepper to taste

For the lasagna:
- 2 large eggplants, sliced lengthwise into 1/4-inch thick slices
- 2 cups marinara sauce
- 1 cup spinach leaves
- Vegan cheese for topping (optional)

Instructions:

- Turn the oven on to 375°F, or 190°C. Coat a baking dish with oil.

- Place the drained tofu, nutritional yeast, lemon juice, dried oregano, dry basil, salt, and pepper in a food processor. Process in a blender until creamy and smooth, like ricotta cheese.
- Arrange the slices of eggplant on a baking pan. Roast for 15 to 20 minutes, or until tender, in an oven that has been warmed.
- Line the bottom of the baking dish that has been prepared with a thin layer of marinara sauce.
- Cover the sauce with a layer of roasted eggplant pieces.
- Cover the eggplant slices with a layer of tofu ricotta and then a layer of spinach leaves.
- Continue layering until all the ingredients have been utilized, and then top with a layer of marinara sauce.
- Top the lasagna with vegan cheese if you'd like.
- Bake the baking dish for 30 to 35 minutes in a preheated oven covered with aluminum foil.

- Take off the foil and bake the lasagna for a further ten to fifteen minutes, or until the top is bubbling and golden brown.
- Allow the lasagna to cool down for a little while before cutting and serving.

7. Cauliflower Steak with Roasted Vegetables:

Ingredients:

- 1 large head cauliflower
- 2 tablespoons olive oil
- 1 teaspoon garlic powder
- 1 teaspoon smoked paprika
- Salt and pepper to taste
- Assorted vegetables for roasting (such as carrots, bell peppers, zucchini, cherry tomatoes)

Instructions:

- Set the oven temperature to 425°F (220°C). Use parchment paper to line a baking sheet.
- Trim the cauliflower stem, leaving the center whole, and remove the leaves.
- Cut the cauliflower into steaks that are 1 inch thick.
- Combine the olive oil, smoked paprika, garlic powder, salt, and pepper in a small bowl.
- Transfer the cauliflower steaks to the prepared baking sheet by brushing both sides with the olive oil mixture.
- On the baking sheet, arrange the other veggies around the cauliflower steaks.
- Roast the cauliflower for 25 to 30 minutes in a preheated oven, turning it halfway through, or until it's soft and browned.
- Present the cauliflower steaks with roasted veggies.

8. Vegan Lentil Curry with Spinach:

Ingredients:

- 1 cup dry green or brown lentils
- 2 cups vegetable broth
- 1 tablespoon olive oil
- 1 onion, diced
- 2 cloves garlic, minced
- 1 tablespoon curry powder
- 1 teaspoon ground cumin
- 1 teaspoon ground turmeric
- ½ teaspoon ground ginger
- 1 can (14 oz) coconut milk
- 2 cups chopped spinach
- Salt and pepper to taste
- Cooked rice for serving
- Fresh cilantro for garnish (optional)

Instructions:

- After rinsing with cold water, drain the lentils.
- Put the lentils and vegetable broth in a saucepan. After bringing to a boil, simmer the lentils for 20 to 25 minutes, covered, or until they are soft and the liquid has been absorbed.
- Heat the olive oil in a big pan over medium heat. Add minced garlic and chopped onion. Cook for five to seven minutes, or until tender.
- Add the ground ginger, turmeric, cumin, and curry powder. Cook until aromatic, about 2 to 3 minutes more.
- Fill the pan with the cooked lentils and coconut milk. Mix everything together.
- Simmer the curry, stirring now and again, for 5 to 7 minutes, or until it's well thickened and cooked through.
- Add the chopped spinach and let it wilt.
- To taste, add salt and pepper for seasoning.

- Top cooked rice with hot lentil curry.
- If preferred, garnish with fresh cilantro.

9. Portobello Mushroom Burgers with Sweet Potato Fries:

Ingredients:

For the Portobello Mushroom Burgers:
- 4 large portobello mushroom caps
- 2 tablespoons balsamic vinegar
- 2 tablespoons soy sauce or tamari
- 2 cloves garlic, minced
- 2 tablespoons olive oil
- Salt and pepper to taste
- Burger buns
- Lettuce, tomato slices, avocado slices, and other desired toppings

For the Sweet Potato Fries:
- 2 large sweet potatoes, peeled and cut into fries
- 2 tablespoons olive oil
- 1 teaspoon garlic powder
- 1 teaspoon paprika
- Salt and pepper to taste

Instructions:

- Set oven temperature to 400°F, or 200°C. Use parchment paper to line a baking sheet.
- Combine the olive oil, soy sauce, minced garlic, balsamic vinegar, salt, and pepper in a bowl. The portobello mushroom caps should be placed in the bowl and covered with marinade. Give them 15 to 20 minutes to marinade.
- In the meanwhile, combine the sweet potato fries with salt, pepper, paprika, garlic powder, and olive oil in another dish and toss until well coated.
- Arrange the sweet potato fries and marinated portobello mushroom caps in a

single layer on the baking sheet that has been ready.
- Bake for 20 to 25 minutes in a preheated oven, rotating the dish halfway through, or until the sweet potato fries are crispy and golden brown and the mushrooms are soft.
- To assemble the burgers, top each bun with a portobello mushroom cap, lettuce, tomato, avocado, and any other toppings you like.

10. Spaghetti Squash with Lentil Bolognese:

Ingredients:

- 1 large spaghetti squash
- 1 tablespoon olive oil
- 1 onion, diced
- 2 cloves garlic, minced
- 1 carrot, diced
- 1 celery stalk, diced
- 1 cup cooked green or brown lentils

- 1 can (14 oz) crushed tomatoes
- 1 teaspoon dried oregano
- 1 teaspoon dried basil
- Salt and pepper to taste
- Fresh basil leaves for garnish (optional)

Instructions:

- Set oven temperature to 400°F, or 200°C.
- Scoop out the seeds after cutting the spaghetti squash in half lengthwise. Spoon the cut side of the squash halves onto a parchment paper-lined baking sheet.
- Bake for 35 to 45 minutes, or until a fork can easily penetrate the squash, in a preheated oven. Take it out of the oven and let it cool a little.
- In a pan over medium heat, warm the olive oil while the squash bakes. Add the chopped carrot, diced celery, minced garlic, and diced onion. Cook for five to seven minutes, or until tender.
- Add the cooked lentils, smashed tomatoes, salt, pepper, dried basil, and dried oregano.

Allow the flavors to merge together by simmering for ten to fifteen minutes, stirring from time to time.
- Scrape the cooked spaghetti squash strands into a big basin using a fork.
- Present the spaghetti squash with bolognese sauce made from lentils on top.
- If preferred, garnish with fresh basil leaves.

11. Vegan Quinoa Fried Rice with Tofu:

Ingredients:

- 1 cup quinoa, rinsed
- 2 cups water or vegetable broth
- 1 tablespoon sesame oil
- 1 block (14 oz) extra-firm tofu, pressed and cubed
- 2 tablespoons soy sauce or tamari
- 1 tablespoon olive oil
- 1 onion, diced

- 2 cloves garlic, minced
- 1 cup mixed vegetables (such as bell peppers, carrots, peas, corn)
- 2 green onions, chopped (for garnish)
- Sesame seeds (for garnish)

Instructions:

- Quinoa should be combined with water or vegetable broth in a saucepan. After bringing to a boil, lower the heat to a simmer, cover, and cook the quinoa for 15 to 20 minutes, or until it is tender and the liquid has been absorbed.
- In a large pan or wok, heat the sesame oil over medium heat while the quinoa cooks. Stir in tamari or soy sauce and cubed tofu. Cook the tofu until it becomes crispy and golden brown on both sides. Take out and place aside from the skillet.
- Heat the olive oil in the same skillet over medium heat. Add minced garlic and chopped onion. Cook for 3–4 minutes, or until tender.

- Add the cooked quinoa and mixed veggies. Cook the veggies for a further five to seven minutes, or until they are crisp-tender.
- Add the cooked tofu back to the pan and stir everything until it is well heated.
- Garnish the hot vegan quinoa fried rice with sesame seeds and chopped green onions.

12. Black Bean Soup with Avocado Salsa:

Ingredients:

For the Black Bean Soup:
- 2 tablespoons olive oil
- 1 onion, diced
- 2 cloves garlic, minced
- 2 cans (15 oz each) black beans, drained and rinsed
- 4 cups vegetable broth
- 1 teaspoon ground cumin
- 1 teaspoon chili powder

- Salt and pepper to taste
- Juice of 1 lime

For the Avocado Salsa:
- 1 ripe avocado, diced
- 1 tomato, diced
- ¼ cup diced red onion
- ¼ cup chopped fresh cilantro
- Juice of 1 lime
- Salt and pepper to taste

Instructions:

- Warm up the olive oil in a big saucepan over medium heat. Add minced garlic and chopped onion. Cook for five to seven minutes, or until tender.
- Add the chili powder, ground cumin, black beans, vegetable broth, salt, and pepper. Simmer for a minimum of 15 to 20 minutes.
- Blend the soup until it's smooth and creamy using an immersion blender. Or put the soup in a blender and process in batches until smooth.

- Add the lime juice and taste and adjust the spice.
- To prepare the avocado salsa, place the diced avocado, diced tomato, diced red onion, chopped fresh cilantro, lime juice, salt, and pepper in a small bowl.
- Ladle a dollop of avocado salsa over the steaming black bean soup.

Snack Recipes

1. Edamame (Steamed Soybeans):

Ingredients:

- 2 cups frozen edamame (shelled)
- 1 tablespoon sea salt (optional)

Instructions:

- In a saucepan, bring the water to a boil.
- Fill the boiling water with the frozen edamame.
- Boil the edamame for four to five minutes, or until they are soft and thoroughly cooked.
- To end the cooking process, drain the edamame and give it a quick rinse with cold water.
- If preferred, top with sea salt.
- As a wholesome snack, serve the edamame warm or cold.

2. Hummus with Sliced Vegetables (Carrots, Cucumber, Bell Peppers):

Ingredients:

- 1 can (15 oz) chickpeas, drained and rinsed
- 2 tablespoons tahini
- 2 tablespoons lemon juice
- 1 clove garlic, minced
- 2 tablespoons olive oil
- Salt and pepper to taste
- Assorted vegetables for dipping (carrot sticks, cucumber slices, bell pepper strips)

Instructions:

- Chickpeas, tahini, lemon juice, minced garlic, olive oil, salt, and pepper should all be combined in a food processor.
- Blend until creamy and smooth, adding a little water as necessary to get the right consistency.
- Spoon the hummus into a dish for serving.

- Spoon the mixed veggies around the hummus bowl on a dish.
- Present the hummus with cut veggies for a dip.

3. Roasted Chickpeas:

Ingredients:

- 1 can (15 oz) chickpeas, drained and rinsed
- 1 tablespoon olive oil
- 1 teaspoon ground cumin
- 1 teaspoon paprika
- 1/2 teaspoon garlic powder
- Salt and pepper to taste

Instructions:

- Set oven temperature to 400°F, or 200°C. Use parchment paper to line a baking sheet.
- Using a paper towel, pat the chickpeas dry to eliminate any remaining moisture.

- Combine the chickpeas, salt, pepper, paprika, ground cumin, and garlic powder in a bowl and toss until well coated.
- Arrange the seasoned chickpeas on the baking sheet that has been preheated in a single layer.
- Bake for 20 to 25 minutes in a preheated oven, stirring the pan halfway through, or until the chickpeas are crispy and golden brown.
- Take it out of the oven and give it a little time to cool before serving.

4. Almond Butter on Whole Grain Crackers:

Ingredients:
- Whole grain crackers
- Almond butter

Instructions:

- Drizzle a large amount of almond butter over whole grain crackers.
- Serve right away as a filling and healthy snack.

5. Vegan Yogurt with Mixed Nuts and Seeds:

Ingredients:

- Vegan yogurt (unsweetened)
- Mixed nuts and seeds (such as almonds, walnuts, pumpkin seeds, sunflower seeds)

Instructions:

- Pour the plant-based yogurt into a bowl.
- Top the yogurt with a mixture of nuts and seeds.
- For a high-protein snack, pair the creamy yogurt with crunchy nuts and seeds.

6. Tofu Salad Wraps in Lettuce Leaves:

Ingredients:

- 1 block (14 oz) extra-firm tofu, pressed and diced
- 1 tablespoon olive oil
- 1 teaspoon garlic powder
- 1 teaspoon onion powder
- ½ teaspoon smoked paprika
- Salt and pepper to taste
- Lettuce leaves (such as romaine or butter lettuce)
- Sliced vegetables (such as bell peppers, cucumbers, carrots)
- Avocado slices (optional)
- Hummus or tahini dressing (optional)

Instructions:

- Heat the olive oil in a pan over medium heat.
- Include the chopped tofu in the pan and season with salt, pepper, smoky paprika, onion powder, and garlic powder.
- Cook for 8 to 10 minutes, or until tofu is crispy and golden brown on both sides.
- Arrange the leaves of lettuce on a dish.
- Transfer tofu onto every leaf of lettuce.
- If desired, add avocado slices and cut veggies on top.
- If using, drizzle with tahini dressing or hummus.
- To make lettuce wraps, roll up the leaves.
- When ready to eat, serve right away or store in the refrigerator.

7. Chia Pudding with Berries:

Ingredients:

- ¼ cup chia seeds
- 1 cup almond milk (or any plant-based milk)
- 1 tablespoon maple syrup or sweetener of choice
- ½ teaspoon vanilla extract
- Mixed berries (such as strawberries, blueberries, raspberries)
- Optional toppings: sliced almonds, shredded coconut, mint leaves

Instructions:

- Chia seeds, almond milk, maple syrup, and vanilla essence should all be combined in a bowl.
- To avoid clumping, let the mixture settle for five minutes before whisking it once more.

- To make the chia pudding thicker, cover the bowl and place it in the refrigerator for at least two hours or overnight.
- To guarantee a uniform consistency, mix the chia pudding just before serving.
- Ladle the chia pudding into dishes or serving cups.
- Add any desired toppings and a mixture of berries over top.
- Serve cold.

8. Vegan Protein Smoothie with Spinach and Almond Milk:

Ingredients:

- 1 cup almond milk
- 1 ripe banana
- 1 cup fresh spinach leaves
- ½ cup silken tofu
- 1 tablespoon almond butter or peanut butter
- 1 tablespoon chia seeds or flaxseeds

- 1 tablespoon hemp seeds (optional)
- Ice cubes (optional)

Instructions:

- Almond milk, ripe banana, fresh spinach leaves, silken tofu, almond butter, chia seeds, and hemp seeds should all be combined in a blender.
- Blend until creamy and smooth.
- If you want a cooler consistency, add ice cubes and mix one more until smooth.
- Transfer the smoothie into cups and start serving right away.

9. Pumpkin Seeds (Pepitas):

Ingredients:

- Raw pumpkin seeds (pepitas)

Instructions:

- Set the oven temperature to 300°F, or 150°C.
- Arrange the raw pumpkin seeds on a baking sheet in a single layer.
- Bake, stirring periodically, in the preheated oven for 15 to 20 minutes, or until the pumpkin seeds are crisp and faintly brown.
- Take it out of the oven, then let it cool down before serving.
- You may eat the roasted pumpkin seeds by themselves as a crisp snack or you can add them to oats, yogurt, and salads.

10. Guacamole with Whole Grain Tortilla Chips:

Ingredients:

- 2 ripe avocados
- 1 small tomato, diced
- ¼ cup diced red onion
- 1 clove garlic, minced
- Juice of 1 lime
- Salt and pepper to taste
- Whole grain tortilla chips

Instructions:

- Remove the pits from the avocados, cut them in half, and scoop out the meat into a dish.
- Using a fork, mash the avocado until it's smooth or chunky, as desired.
- Until fully blended, stir in chopped tomato, diced red onion, minced garlic, lime juice, salt, and pepper.

- Taste and, if necessary, adjust the seasoning.
- Offer healthy grain tortilla chips for dipping with the guacamole.

Dessert Recipes

1. Vegan Chocolate Avocado Mousse:

Ingredients:

- 2 ripe avocados
- ¼ cup cocoa powder
- ¼ cup maple syrup or sweetener of choice
- 1 teaspoon vanilla extract
- Pinch of salt
- Optional toppings: sliced strawberries, raspberries, shredded coconut

Instructions:

- Halve the avocados, remove the pits, and transfer the flesh to a blender or food processor.
- Fill the blender with cocoa powder, vanilla extract, maple syrup, and a dash of salt.
- Blend until everything is fully blended, scraping down the sides as necessary, until the mixture is smooth and creamy.

- Spoon the mousse made of chocolate and avocado into glasses or serving bowls.
- Chill and put in the refrigerator for at least 30 minutes.
- Top with shredded coconut, strawberries, or raspberries, if you'd like.

2. Chickpea Blondies:

Ingredients:

- 1 can (15 oz) chickpeas, drained and rinsed
- ½ cup almond butter or peanut butter
- ¼ cup maple syrup or sweetener of choice
- 1 teaspoon vanilla extract
- ½ teaspoon baking powder
- Pinch of salt
- ¼ cup vegan chocolate chips (optional)

Instructions:

- Set the oven's temperature to 175°C/350°F. Line a baking dish with parchment paper or grease it.
- Put the chickpeas, almond butter, maple syrup, baking powder, vanilla extract, and a little amount of salt in a food processor.
- Blend, scraping down the sides as necessary, until creamy and smooth.
- Add vegan chocolate chips, if using, and fold until they are spread evenly.
- Evenly spread out the chickpea blondie batter in the baking dish that has been prepared.
- Bake for 20 to 25 minutes in a preheated oven, or until a toothpick inserted into the middle comes out clean and the sides are golden brown.
- Take out of the oven, let cool, then cut into squares.

3. Almond Flour Cookies:

Ingredients:

- 2 cups almond flour
- ¼ cup maple syrup or sweetener of choice
- ¼ cup coconut oil, melted
- 1 teaspoon vanilla extract
- Pinch of salt
- Optional add-ins: vegan chocolate chips, chopped nuts, dried fruit

Instructions:

- Set the oven's temperature to 175°C/350°F. Use parchment paper to line a baking sheet.
- Place almond flour, maple syrup, melted coconut oil, vanilla essence, and a little amount of salt in a mixing dish.
- Stir until a dense dough for cookies forms.
- Gently stir in dried fruit, chopped nuts, or vegan chocolate chips, if using, until everything is spread equally.

- Divide the dough into equal halves and form it into balls using a spoon or cookie scoop.
- Transfer the dough balls to the baking sheet that has been prepared, and use your hand to gently flatten them.
- Bake for 10 to 12 minutes, or until the edges of the cookies are golden brown, in a preheated oven.
- Take out of the oven and let it rest for a few minutes on the baking sheet, then place it on a wire rack to cool down entirely.

4. Peanut Butter Banana Nice Cream:

Ingredients:

- 3 ripe bananas, sliced and frozen
- 2 tablespoons peanut butter
- ¼ cup almond milk or any plant-based milk
- Optional toppings: chopped peanuts, vegan chocolate chips, sliced bananas

Instructions:

- In a food processor or blender, combine the frozen banana slices, peanut butter, and almond milk.
- Blend, scraping down the sides as necessary, until creamy and smooth.
- Add more almond milk, one tablespoon at a time, to the lovely cream if it's too thick, until you have the right consistency.
- Spoon the excellent cream with peanut butter and banana into serving dishes.
- Top with sliced bananas, vegan chocolate chips, or chopped peanuts and serve right away.

5. Baked Apples with Cinnamon and Walnuts:

Ingredients:

- 4 apples (such as Granny Smith or Honeycrisp)
- ¼ cup chopped walnuts
- 2 tablespoons maple syrup or sweetener of choice
- 1 teaspoon ground cinnamon
- Pinch of nutmeg (optional)
- Pinch of salt
- Vegan butter or coconut oil (for greasing)

Instructions:

- Turn the oven on to 375°F, or 190°C. Use coconut oil or vegan butter to grease a baking dish.
- After coring the apples, cut them into ½-inch-thick horizontal rings.
- Put the apple slices in the baking dish that has been prepared in a single layer.

- Place chopped walnuts, maple syrup, ground cinnamon, nutmeg (if using), and a little amount of salt in a small bowl.
- Fill the middle where the core was by spooning the walnut mixture over each apple slice.
- Bake the baking dish in the preheated oven for 20 to 25 minutes, or until the apples are soft, covered with foil.
- Take it out of the oven and give it a little time to cool before serving.

6. Protein-Rich Vegan Brownies:

Ingredients:

- 1 can (15 oz) black beans, drained and rinsed
- ½ cup cocoa powder
- ½ cup almond butter or peanut butter
- ¼ cup maple syrup or sweetener of choice
- 1 teaspoon vanilla extract
- ½ teaspoon baking powder

- Pinch of salt
- Vegan chocolate chips (optional)

Instructions:

- Set the oven's temperature to 175°C/350°F. Line a baking dish with parchment paper or grease it.
- Put almond butter, maple syrup, baking powder, cocoa powder, black beans, vanilla essence, and a little amount of salt in a food processor.
- Blend, scraping down the sides as necessary, until creamy and smooth.
- Add vegan chocolate chips, if using, and fold until they are spread evenly.
- Evenly spread out the brownie batter after pouring it onto the baking dish that has been prepared.
- Bake for 25 to 30 minutes in a preheated oven, or until the toothpick inserted into the middle comes out clean and the sides are firm.

- Take out of the oven, let cool, then cut into squares.

7. Coconut Yogurt Parfait with Berries:

Ingredients:

- 1 cup coconut yogurt (unsweetened)
- ½ cup mixed berries (such as strawberries, blueberries, raspberries)
- ¼ cup granola
- Optional toppings: shredded coconut, sliced almonds, drizzle of maple syrup

Instructions:

- Arrange granola, mixed berries, and coconut yogurt in a serving dish or glass.
- Continue layering until the bowl or glass is full.

- If preferred, garnish with sliced almonds, shredded coconut, and maple syrup.
- Serve the coconut yogurt parfait with berries.

8. Quinoa Chocolate Bark with Nuts and Seeds:

Ingredients:

- ½ cup cooked quinoa
- ½ cup vegan chocolate chips
- 2 tablespoons chopped nuts (such as almonds, walnuts, pecans)
- 2 tablespoons mixed seeds (such as pumpkin seeds, sunflower seeds)
- Pinch of sea salt

Instructions:

- Use parchment paper to line a baking sheet.

- Evenly distribute the cooked quinoa onto the parchment paper.
- Melt vegan chocolate chips in a microwave-safe dish for 30 seconds at a time, or until they are smooth and creamy.
- Using a spatula, evenly distribute the melted chocolate over the cooked quinoa.
- Top the melted chocolate with chopped nuts, mixed seeds, and a dash of sea salt.
- Refrigerate the baking sheet for one to two hours, or until the chocolate bark sets.
- Break the chocolate bark into pieces when it has hardened.

9. Tofu Cheesecake Bites:

Ingredients:

- 1 block (14 oz) firm tofu, drained
- ¼ cup maple syrup or sweetener of choice
- ¼ cup lemon juice
- 1 teaspoon vanilla extract

- ¼ cup coconut oil, melted
- Pinch of salt
- Graham cracker crumbs (for crust, optional)
- Mixed berries (for topping, optional)

Instructions:

- Melted coconut oil, lemon juice, vanilla extract, firm tofu, maple syrup, and a dash of salt should all be combined in a food processor or blender.
- Blend, scraping down the sides as necessary, until creamy and smooth.
- To create a crust, if using, press graham cracker crumbs into the bottom of mini muffin liners.
- Almost to the top, spoon the tofu cheesecake mixture into the small muffin liners.
- Chill the tofu cheesecake pieces in the fridge for at least two hours, or until they solidify.

- Take the tofu cheesecake bites out of the muffin liners after they have set.
- If preferred, sprinkle mixed berries on top.

10. Vegan Protein Pancakes with Berries:

Ingredients:

- 1 cup all-purpose flour or whole wheat flour
- ¼ cup vegan protein powder
- 1 tablespoon baking powder
- 1 tablespoon coconut sugar or maple syrup
- 1 cup plant-based milk (such as almond milk or soy milk)
- 2 tablespoons melted coconut oil or vegetable oil
- 1 teaspoon vanilla extract
- 1 cup mixed berries (such as strawberries, blueberries, raspberries)
- Maple syrup for serving (optional)

Instructions:

- Mix the flour, coconut sugar, baking powder, and vegan protein powder in a big bowl.
- Combine the melted coconut oil, vanilla extract, and plant-based milk with the dry ingredients. Take care not to overmix; stir just until incorporated.
- Turn up the heat to medium on a nonstick skillet or griddle. For each pancake, add ¼ cup of batter to the skillet.
- Cook the pancakes until bubbles appear on their top, then turn them over and cook the second side until golden brown.
- If wanted, top the vegan protein pancakes with maple syrup and a mixture of fruit.

11. Oatmeal Raisin Cookies with Walnuts:

Ingredients:

- 1 cup rolled oats
- ¾ cup whole wheat flour or all-purpose flour
- ½ teaspoon baking soda
- ½ teaspoon ground cinnamon
- ¼ teaspoon salt
- ¼ cup melted coconut oil or vegetable oil
- ¼ cup maple syrup or coconut sugar
- ¼ cup unsweetened applesauce
- 1 teaspoon vanilla extract
- ½ cup raisins
- ¼ cup chopped walnuts

Instructions:

- Set the oven's temperature to 175°C/350°F. Use parchment paper to line a baking sheet.

- Mix the flour, baking soda, cinnamon, salt, and rolled oats in a large basin.

- Combine the applesauce, vanilla extract, maple syrup, and melted coconut oil in another bowl.

- After adding the wet components to the dry ingredients, whisk everything together well.

- Add the chopped walnuts and raisins and fold.

- Drop dough spoonfuls, approximately two inches apart, onto the baking sheet that has been prepared.

- Using the back of a spoon, gently flatten the dough.

- Bake the cookies for ten to twelve minutes, or until they are golden brown.

- Take out of the oven and let it rest for a few minutes on the baking sheet, then place it on a wire rack to cool down entirely.

12. Berry Smoothie Bowl with Granola:

Ingredients:

- 1 frozen banana, sliced
- 1 cup mixed berries (such as strawberries, blueberries, raspberries)
- ½ cup plant-based milk (such as almond milk or coconut milk)
- 1 tablespoon chia seeds (optional)
- ¼ cup granola
- Fresh berries and sliced banana for topping

Instructions:

- Blend together the frozen banana, plant-based milk, mixed berries, and chia seeds, if desired, using a blender. Blend till creamy and smooth.
- Transfer the blended drink to a basin.
- Add granola, banana slices, and fresh berries over top.

13. Protein-Packed Vegan Truffles:

Ingredients:

- 1 cup pitted dates
- ½ cup almonds
- ¼ cup cocoa powder
- 2 tablespoons vegan protein powder
- 1 tablespoon maple syrup
- Pinch of salt
- Shredded coconut, cocoa powder, or crushed nuts for rolling (optional)

Instructions:

- Pitted dates, almonds, vegan protein powder, maple syrup, cocoa powder, and a dash of salt should all be combined in a food processor.
- Process until a sticky dough is formed from the ingredients.
- Form the dough into little spheres.

- For added taste and texture, you may optionally roll the truffles in chopped almonds, cocoa powder, or shredded coconut.
- Before serving, place the truffles in the fridge to cool for at least half an hour.

14. Coconut Flour Banana Bread:

Ingredients:

- 3 ripe bananas, mashed
- ¼ cup melted coconut oil or vegetable oil
- ¼ cup maple syrup or coconut sugar
- 3 tablespoons plant-based milk (such as almond milk or soy milk)
- 1 teaspoon vanilla extract
- ¾ cup coconut flour
- 1 teaspoon baking powder
- ½ teaspoon baking soda
- Pinch of salt
- ½ cup chopped walnuts (optional)

Instructions:

- Set the oven's temperature to 175°C/350°F. Line a 9x5-inch loaf pan with parchment paper or grease it.
- Put the mashed bananas, plant-based milk, maple syrup, melted coconut oil, and vanilla extract in a big bowl.
- Combine the coconut flour, baking soda, baking powder, and salt in another basin.
- Stir just until well blended after adding the dry ingredients to the wet ones.
- If using, fold in the chopped walnuts.
- Transfer the mixture into the loaf pan that has been ready and use a spatula to level the top.
Bake for forty-five to fifty minutes, or until a toothpick inserted in the middle comes out clean.
- Take out of the oven and let it cool in the pan for ten minutes, then place it on a wire rack to finish cooling.

15. Vegan Protein Ice Cream with Almond Milk:

Ingredients:

- 2 ripe bananas, sliced and frozen
- 1 cup unsweetened almond milk
- 2 tablespoons vegan protein powder
- 1 tablespoon maple syrup or coconut sugar
- 1 teaspoon vanilla extract

Instructions:

- The frozen banana slices, almond milk, vegan protein powder, maple syrup, and vanilla extract should all be combined in a blender.
- Blend until creamy and smooth, stopping the blender as necessary to scrape down the sides.
- To avoid ice crystals developing, transfer the mixture to a shallow dish and freeze for two to three hours, stirring every thirty minutes.

- Serve the ice cream in dishes or cones after it's solid but still scoopable.

Quick and Easy Recipes for Busy Moms

1. Lentil Soup:

Ingredients:

- 1 cup dried lentils
- 4 cups vegetable broth
- 1 onion, diced
- 2 carrots, diced
- 2 celery stalks, diced
- 2 cloves garlic, minced
- 1 teaspoon ground cumin
- 1 teaspoon paprika
- Salt and pepper to taste
- Fresh parsley for garnish (optional)

Instructions:

- After rinsing with cold water, drain the lentils.
- Heat a little amount of oil in a big saucepan over medium heat. Add the celery,

carrots, and chopped onion. Simmer for approximately 5 minutes, or until tender.
- Include the paprika, ground cumin, and chopped garlic. Cook until aromatic, about 1 more minute.
- Fill the pot with the lentils and vegetable broth. After bringing to a boil, lower the heat and simmer the lentils for 20 to 25 minutes, or until they are soft.
- To taste, add salt and pepper for seasoning.
- Garnish with fresh parsley, if preferred, and serve hot.

2. Chickpea Salad Wraps:

Ingredients:

- 1 can (15 oz) chickpeas, drained and rinsed
- ¼ cup diced red onion
- ¼ cup diced cucumber
- ¼ cup diced bell pepper

- 2 tablespoons chopped fresh parsley
- Juice of 1 lemon
- Salt and pepper to taste
- Whole grain wraps or lettuce leaves for serving

Instructions:

- Using a fork, gently mash the chickpeas in a bowl.
- Include the bell pepper, sliced red onion, cucumber, chopped parsley, lemon juice, salt, and pepper. Toss to blend thoroughly.
- Transfer the chickpea salad on lettuce leaves or whole grain wrappers.
- To construct wraps, roll up the lettuce leaves or wraps.
- When ready to eat, serve right away or store in the refrigerator.

3. Vegan Chili:

Ingredients:

- 1 tablespoon olive oil
- 1 onion, diced
- 2 cloves garlic, minced
- 1 bell pepper, diced
- 1 zucchini, diced
- 1 can (15 oz) diced tomatoes
- 1 can (15 oz) kidney beans, drained and rinsed
- 1 can (15 oz) black beans, drained and rinsed
- 2 cups vegetable broth
- 2 tablespoons chili powder
- 1 teaspoon cumin
- Salt and pepper to taste
- Optional toppings: diced avocado, chopped cilantro, vegan sour cream

Instructions:

- In a big saucepan, warm up the olive oil over medium heat. Add minced garlic and chopped onion. Simmer for five minutes, or until tender.
- Include the pot with the chopped bell pepper and zucchini. Cook until the veggies are soft, about 5 more minutes.
- Add the chopped tomatoes, cumin, chili powder, black beans, kidney beans, and vegetable broth.
- Simmer the chili for 20 to 25 minutes, stirring from time to time, before lowering the heat.
- Taste and adjust the seasoning if necessary.
- Top with chopped cilantro, sliced avocado, and vegan sour cream, if preferred, and serve hot.

4. Avocado and White Bean Wraps:

Ingredients:

- 1 ripe avocado
- 1 can (15 oz) white beans, drained and rinsed
- ¼ cup diced red onion
- ¼ cup chopped fresh cilantro
- Juice of 1 lime
- Salt and pepper to taste
- 4 whole grain wraps or lettuce leaves

Instructions:

- Mash the white beans with a fork in a bowl.
- To the mashed beans, add sliced red onion, chopped cilantro, lime juice, salt, and pepper. Blend well.
- Mound each lettuce leaf or wrap with mashed avocado.
- Top the avocado with a spoonful of the white bean mixture.

- After rolling the lettuce leaves or wraps, serve.

5. Eggplant Stir-Fry with Brown Rice:

Ingredients:

- 1 large eggplant, diced
- 2 cups mixed vegetables (bell peppers, broccoli, carrots)
- 2 tablespoons soy sauce
- 1 tablespoon sesame oil
- 2 cloves garlic, minced
- Cooked brown rice for serving
- Optional garnish: chopped green onions, sesame seeds

Instructions:

- In a big skillet or wok, warm up the sesame oil over medium heat.

- Cook the minced garlic in the pan for one minute.
- Fill the pan with chopped eggplant and other veggies. Vegetables should be stir-fried for 5 to 7 minutes to soften them.
- Cook for a further two to three minutes after adding the soy sauce.
- Arrange the cooked brown rice on top of the stir-fried eggplant.
- If preferred, garnish with sesame seeds and chopped green onions.

6. Vegan Burrito Bowls:

Ingredients:

- 1 cup cooked brown rice or quinoa
- 1 can (15 oz) black beans, drained and rinsed
- 1 cup corn kernels (fresh or frozen)
- 1 cup diced tomatoes
- 1 avocado, diced
- ¼ cup diced red onion

- ¼ cup chopped fresh cilantro
- Juice of 1 lime
- Salt and pepper to taste

Instructions:

- Spoon cooked quinoa or brown rice into individual serving dishes.
- Add chopped cilantro, diced red onion, diced avocado, diced tomatoes, black beans, and corn kernels on top.
- Add salt and pepper to the bowls and drizzle with lime juice.
- Present the plant-based burrito bowls right away.

7. Vegan Protein Smoothies with Leafy Greens:

Ingredients:

- 1 cup unsweetened almond milk
- 1 ripe banana

- 1 cup fresh spinach or kale leaves
- ½ cup frozen mixed berries
- 1 tablespoon chia seeds or flaxseeds
- 1 scoop vegan protein powder (optional)
- Ice cubes (optional)

Instructions:

- Blend together unsweetened almond milk, ripe banana, frozen mixed berries, fresh spinach or kale leaves, chia or flax seeds, and vegan protein powder, if using, in a blender.
- Blend until creamy and smooth.
- Blend again until smooth, adding ice cubes if a cooler consistency is preferred.
- Transfer the smoothie into cups and start serving right away.

Flavorful Vegan Meals to Satisfy Every Palate

1. Vegan Teriyaki Tofu Stir-Fry:

Ingredients:

- 1 block (14 oz) tofu, pressed and cubed
- 2 tablespoons soy sauce
- 2 tablespoons teriyaki sauce
- 1 tablespoon maple syrup or agave nectar
- 1 tablespoon sesame oil
- 2 cloves garlic, minced
- 1 teaspoon grated ginger
- 2 cups mixed vegetables (bell peppers, broccoli, carrots)
- Cooked rice or noodles for serving

Instructions:

- Combine the soy sauce, teriyaki sauce, maple syrup, sesame oil, grated ginger, and chopped garlic in a bowl.

- For at least fifteen minutes, marinate the cubed tofu in the sauce mixture.
- Turn up the heat to medium in a big wok or pan. When the tofu has marinated, add it and fry it till golden brown all over.
- Put the mixed veggies in the pan and stir-fry them until they are crisp-tender.
- Top cooked rice or noodles with the teriyaki tofu and veggies.

2. Zucchini Noodles with Lentil Marinara Sauce:

Ingredients:

- 2 large zucchinis, spiralized into noodles
- 1 can (15 oz) lentils, drained and rinsed
- 2 cups marinara sauce
- 2 cloves garlic, minced
- 1 tablespoon olive oil
- Salt and pepper to taste
- Fresh basil leaves for garnish

Instructions:

- In a big skillet over medium heat, warm up the olive oil. When aromatic, add the minced garlic and simmer.
- Cook the spiralized zucchini noodles in the pan for 3–4 minutes, or until they are soft.
- Add marinara sauce and lentils and stir. Cook until well heated.
- To taste, add salt and pepper for seasoning.
- Garnish the zucchini noodles with fresh basil leaves and serve them with lentil marinara sauce.

3. Vegan Taco Salad with Walnut Meat:

Ingredients:

For Walnut Meat:
- 1 cup walnuts
- 1 tablespoon chili powder
- 1 teaspoon ground cumin
- ½ teaspoon paprika
- Salt and pepper to taste

For Salad:
- Mixed salad greens
- Cherry tomatoes, halved
- Sliced avocado
- Black beans, drained and rinsed
- Corn kernels (fresh or frozen)
- Sliced red onion
- Salsa for dressing

Instructions:

- Pulse walnuts in a food processor until finely chopped.
- Fill the food processor with the ground cumin, paprika, chili powder, salt, and pepper. Pulse until thoroughly mixed.
- Turn up the heat to medium in a skillet. Stir in walnut mixture and heat for 5 to 7 minutes, or until aromatic and gently browned. Take off the heat and put it aside.
- In a big bowl, combine salad greens, cherry tomatoes, black beans, corn kernels, sliced avocado, and sliced red onion.
- Add walnut meat to the salad.
- As a dressing, drizzle salsa over the salad.
- Combine with a toss and serve right away.

4. Stuffed Acorn Squash with Wild Rice and Cranberries:

Ingredients:
- 2 acorn squashes, halved and seeds removed
- 1 cup wild rice, cooked
- ½ cup dried cranberries
- ¼ cup chopped pecans
- 2 tablespoons maple syrup
- 1 tablespoon olive oil
- Salt and pepper to taste

Instructions:

- Set oven temperature to 400°F, or 200°C.
- Cut side up, arrange the acorn squash halves on a baking sheet.
- Combine cooked wild rice, chopped nuts, dried cranberries, maple syrup, olive oil, salt, and pepper in a bowl.
- Fill the halves of the acorn squash with the rice mixture.

- Bake the squash for 40 to 45 minutes, or until it is soft, covered with foil on the baking sheet.
- Take out of the oven and present it warm.

5. Vegan Mediterranean Stuffed Peppers:

Ingredients:

- 4 bell peppers, halved and seeds removed
- 1 cup cooked quinoa
- 1 can (15 oz) chickpeas, drained and rinsed
- ½ cup chopped cherry tomatoes
- ¼ cup diced red onion
- ¼ cup chopped fresh parsley
- 2 tablespoons lemon juice
- 2 tablespoons olive oil
- Salt and pepper to taste

Instructions:

- Turn the oven on to 375°F, or 190°C.
- Lay out the bell pepper halves, cut side up, on a baking sheet.
- Combine cooked quinoa, chickpeas, diced red onion, chopped cherry tomatoes, chopped fresh parsley, lemon juice, olive oil, salt, and pepper in a bowl.
- Fill the bell pepper halves with the quinoa mixture using a spoon.
- Bake the peppers for 25 to 30 minutes, or until they are soft, while covering the baking sheet with foil.
- Take out of the oven and present it warm.

6. Thai Coconut Curry Noodles with Vegetables:

Ingredients:

- 8 oz rice noodles
- 1 tablespoon coconut oil

- 1 small onion, thinly sliced
- 2 cloves garlic, minced
- 1 red bell pepper, thinly sliced
- 1 carrot, julienned
- 1 cup broccoli florets
- 1 can (14 oz) coconut milk
- 2 tablespoons Thai red curry paste
- 2 tablespoons soy sauce or tamari
- 1 tablespoon maple syrup or coconut sugar
- Juice of 1 lime
- Salt to taste
- Fresh cilantro and lime wedges for garnish

Instructions:

- Follow the directions on the box to cook the rice noodles. After draining, put away.
- Heat the coconut oil in a big pan or wok over medium heat. Add the minced garlic and chopped onion. Cook for two to three minutes, or until tender.
- Include the broccoli florets, julienned carrot, and sliced red bell pepper in the pan.

Stir-fry the veggies for 3–4 minutes, or until they are crisp-tender.

- Combine the coconut milk, soy sauce, lime juice, Thai red curry paste, and maple syrup in a small bowl.

- Cover the veggies in the pan with the curry sauce. Simmer and cook for two to three minutes.

Toss the cooked rice noodles with the curry sauce in the pan once they have been cooked.

- Add salt to taste for seasoning.

- Garnish the hot Thai coconut curry noodles with lime wedges and chopped cilantro.

7. Vegan Butternut Squash Soup with Coconut Milk:

Ingredients:

- 1 medium butternut squash, peeled, seeded, and diced

- 1 tablespoon olive oil
- 1 onion, chopped
- 2 cloves garlic, minced
- 1 teaspoon ground cumin
- ½ teaspoon ground cinnamon
- ¼ teaspoon ground nutmeg
- 4 cups vegetable broth
- 1 can (14 oz) coconut milk
- Salt and pepper to taste
- Toasted pumpkin seeds for garnish (optional)
- Fresh parsley or cilantro for garnish (optional)

Instructions:

- Warm up the olive oil in a big saucepan over medium heat. Add minced garlic and diced onion. Cook for 3–4 minutes, or until tender.

- Fill the saucepan with chopped butternut squash. Cook for another five minutes, stirring now and again.
- Add the ground nutmeg, cinnamon, and cumin and stir. Simmer for one minute, or until aromatic.
- Fill the kettle with vegetable broth. When butternut squash is soft, decrease heat, simmer for 20 to 25 minutes, after bringing to a boil.
- Blend the soup until it's smooth using an immersion blender or a blender.
- Put the pureed soup back in the saucepan. Add coconut milk, stir, and fully cook.
- To taste, add salt and pepper for seasoning.
- Garnish the hot vegan butternut squash soup with toasted pumpkin seeds and, if preferred, fresh parsley or cilantro.

8. Mediterranean Chickpea Salad with Tahini Dressing:

Ingredients:

- 2 cans (15 oz each) chickpeas, drained and rinsed
- 1 cucumber, diced
- 1 cup cherry tomatoes, halved
- ½ red onion, thinly sliced
- ¼ cup chopped fresh parsley
- ¼ cup chopped fresh mint
- ¼ cup pitted Kalamata olives, halved
- Juice of 1 lemon
- 2 tablespoons tahini
- 2 tablespoons olive oil
- 1 clove garlic, minced
- Salt and pepper to taste

Instructions:

- Chickpeas, diced cucumber, half-peeled cherry tomatoes, thinly sliced red onion, chopped fresh parsley, chopped fresh mint,

and half-cut Kalamata olives should all be combined in a big dish.
- To create the dressing, combine the lemon juice, tahini, olive oil, chopped garlic, salt, and pepper in a small bowl.
- Drizzle the chickpea salad with the tahini dressing and toss to cover well.
- You may serve the chilled or room temperature Mediterranean chickpea salad.

9. Vegan Mushroom Stroganoff with Cashew Cream:

Ingredients:

- 8 oz fettuccine or any pasta of choice
- 2 tablespoons olive oil
- 1 onion, chopped
- 2 cloves garlic, minced
- 8 oz cremini mushrooms, sliced
- 1 teaspoon dried thyme
- ¼ cup vegetable broth

- 1 cup cashews, soaked in water for 2 hours or overnight
- 1 cup water
- 2 tablespoons nutritional yeast
- 1 tablespoon lemon juice
- Salt and pepper to taste
- Chopped fresh parsley for garnish

Instructions:

- Follow the directions on the box to cook the fettuccine. After draining, put away.
- Heat the olive oil in a big skillet over medium heat. Add minced garlic and diced onion. Cook for 3–4 minutes, or until tender.
- Fill the pan with cut cremini mushrooms. Cook for 5 to 6 minutes, or until mushrooms are golden brown.
- Add the veggie broth and dried thyme. Cook until well cooked, 2 to 3 minutes more.
- Put the soaked cashews (drained) with water, nutritional yeast, and lemon juice in a blender. Blend till creamy and smooth.

- Add cashew cream to the mushroom-filled skillet. Mix well and warm through.
- To taste, add salt and pepper for seasoning.
- Top the cooked fettuccine with the vegan mushroom stroganoff and sprinkle with fresh parsley.

10. Vegan Pasta Primavera

Ingredients:

- 8 oz pasta (such as spaghetti, fettuccine, or penne)
- 2 tablespoons olive oil
- 3 cloves garlic, minced
- 1 small onion, thinly sliced
- 2 cups mixed vegetables (such as bell peppers, broccoli, carrots, cherry tomatoes, zucchini), chopped
- 1 cup cherry tomatoes, halved
- ½ cup vegetable broth

- ½ cup canned coconut milk
- 1 tablespoon nutritional yeast (optional)
- 1 tablespoon lemon juice
- Salt and pepper to taste
- Fresh basil or parsley for garnish (optional)

Instructions:

- Pasta should be cooked as directed on the box until it is al dente. After draining, put away.
- Heat the olive oil in a big skillet over medium heat. Add the thinly sliced onion and minced garlic. Simmer the onion for 3–4 minutes, or until it is aromatic and transparent.
- Fill the pan with the mixed veggies. Simmer for 5 to 6 minutes, or until they begin to soften.
- Add the cherry tomatoes and simmer for a further two to three minutes.
- Add the coconut milk and vegetable broth. If using, stir with the nutritional yeast. After

bringing to a simmer, cook for two to three minutes.

- Fill the skillet with the cooked pasta. Give the spaghetti a good toss to evenly distribute the sauce and veggies.

- Add the lemon juice and season to taste with salt and pepper.

- Turn off the heat and, if preferred, sprinkle on some fresh parsley or basil.

11. Mexican-Inspired Vegan Quinoa Salad:

Ingredients:

- 1 cup quinoa
- 1½ cups water or vegetable broth
- 1 can (15 oz) black beans, drained and rinsed
- 1 cup corn kernels (fresh or frozen)
- 1 red bell pepper, diced
- ½ red onion, finely chopped

- 1 jalapeño, seeded and minced
- ¼ cup chopped fresh cilantro
- Juice of 2 limes
- 2 tablespoons olive oil
- 1 teaspoon ground cumin
- 1 teaspoon chili powder
- Salt and pepper to taste
- Avocado slices for serving (optional)

Instructions:

- Wash the quinoa in cool water. Bring water or vegetable broth to a boil in a medium-sized pot. When the quinoa is cooked and the water has been absorbed, add it, lower the heat to low, cover it, and simmer it for 15 to 20 minutes. Turn off the heat and let it cool.
- Transfer cooked quinoa, black beans, corn kernels, finely sliced red onion, diced red bell pepper, minced jalapeño, and chopped fresh cilantro into a large mixing dish.

- Combine the lime juice, olive oil, chili powder, powdered cumin, salt, and pepper in a small bowl.
- Drizzle the quinoa salad with the dressing and mix well.
- You can serve the vegan quinoa salad with a Mexican flair at room temperature or chilled. You can even garnish it with avocado slices if you want.

12. Korean-Inspired Tofu Bibimbap Bowls:

Ingredients:

- 1 cup uncooked short-grain white rice
- 1½ cups water
- 1 block (14 oz) extra-firm tofu, pressed and cubed
- 2 tablespoons soy sauce or tamari
- 1 tablespoon sesame oil
- 2 cloves garlic, minced
- 1 tablespoon rice vinegar

- 1 tablespoon maple syrup or agave nectar
- 2 cups mixed vegetables (such as spinach, carrots, bean sprouts, mushrooms)
- 2 tablespoons gochujang (Korean chili paste)
- Sesame seeds for garnish
- Sliced green onions for garnish

Instructions:

- Follow the directions on the box to cook the rice.
- Combine soy sauce, rice vinegar, maple syrup, sesame oil, and chopped garlic in a bowl. Let the cubed tofu marinade for at least fifteen minutes after adding it.
- Turn up the heat to medium in a big skillet. The marinated tofu should be added and cooked until golden brown all over.
- Stir-fry mixed veggies in the same pan until they are crisp-tender.
- Spoon cooked rice into each serving dish to make the bibimbap bowls. Top the rice with the mixed veggies and cooked tofu.

- Top each dish with sliced green onions and sesame seeds, and serve with a dollop of gochujang.
- Combine all ingredients well before consuming.

13. Italian-Inspired Vegan Pasta Primavera:

Ingredients:

- 8 oz pasta (such as spaghetti or fettuccine)
- 2 tablespoons olive oil
- 3 cloves garlic, minced
- 1 small onion, thinly sliced
- 2 cups mixed vegetables (such as bell peppers, cherry tomatoes, zucchini, broccoli)
- ½ cup vegetable broth
- ¼ cup canned coconut milk
- 2 tablespoons nutritional yeast (optional)
- 1 tablespoon lemon juice
- Salt and pepper to taste

- Fresh basil leaves for garnish (optional)

Instructions:

- Cook the pasta according to the package's instructions until it's al dente. After emptying, store.
- In a large pan, warm the olive oil over medium heat. Add the minced garlic and the thinly sliced onion. Cook until tender, 3–4 minutes.
- Arrange a variety of vegetables in the pan. Simmer until they start to become tender, about 5 to 6 minutes.
- Pour the vegetable broth and coconut milk into the skillet. Stir in nutritional yeast, if using. Cook for two to three minutes while simmering.
- Add the cooked pasta to the pan. Toss to coat the pasta in a uniform layer of sauce and vegetables.
- Include the lemon juice and add salt and pepper to taste.

- Taking a cue from Italy, garnish the hot, vegan spaghetti primavera with fresh basil leaves if desired.

14. Middle Eastern-Inspired Falafel with Hummus and Tabouleh:

Ingredients:

- 1 can (15 oz) chickpeas, drained and rinsed
- ¼ cup chopped fresh parsley
- ¼ cup chopped fresh cilantro
- ½ small onion, chopped
- 2 cloves garlic, minced
- 1 teaspoon ground cumin
- 1 teaspoon ground coriander
- ¼ teaspoon cayenne pepper
- Salt and pepper to taste
- 2 tablespoons chickpea flour or all-purpose flour
- 2 tablespoons olive oil for frying
- Hummus for serving

- Tabouleh for serving
- Pita bread or lettuce leaves for serving

Instructions:

- Chickpeas, chopped parsley, chopped cilantro, chopped onion, minced garlic, ground cumin, ground coriander, cayenne pepper, salt, and pepper should all be combined in a food processor. Pulse the mixture until it's thoroughly mixed but has some chunks remaining.
- Spoon the blend into a basin. Add all-purpose or chickpea flour and stir until the mixture comes together.
- Form the mixture into little patties or balls.
- In a pan over medium heat, warm the olive oil. Fry the falafel patties or balls for 3–4 minutes on each side, or until they are crispy and golden brown on both sides.
- Accompany falafel with pita bread or lettuce leaves, hummus, and tabouleh.

15. Jamaican-Inspired Vegan Jerk Tofu with Rice and Beans:

Ingredients:

- 1 block (14 oz) extra-firm tofu, pressed and sliced
- 2 tablespoons Jamaican jerk seasoning
- 2 tablespoons olive oil
- 1 cup uncooked white rice
- 1 can (15 oz) black beans, drained and rinsed
- ¼ cup chopped fresh cilantro for garnish
- Lime wedges for serving

Instructions:

- Tofu should be pressed to eliminate extra water. Cut the tofu into rectangles or cubes.
- Evenly sprinkle the tofu slices with the Jamaican jerk flavor by tossing them in a dish.
- In a pan over medium-high heat, warm the olive oil. When the tofu slices are golden

brown and crispy, add them to the pan and cook for three to four minutes on each side.
- In the meanwhile, prepare the white rice per the directions on the box.
- Bring the black beans to a simmer over medium heat in a different saucepan.
- Take the cooked tofu out of the pan and place it somewhere else.
- Spoon cooked rice onto serving dishes. Place the warmed black beans and cooked tofu pieces on top.
- Serve with lime wedges on the side and garnish with freshly chopped cilantro.
- Savor your vegan jerk tofu with rice and beans.

16. Indian-Inspired Vegan Lentil Dal:

Ingredients:

- 1 cup dried red lentils
- 4 cups water
- 1 tablespoon olive oil or coconut oil
- 1 onion, finely chopped
- 3 cloves garlic, minced
- 1 tablespoon grated ginger
- 1 teaspoon ground turmeric
- 1 teaspoon ground cumin
- 1 teaspoon ground coriander
- ½ teaspoon garam masala
- ¼ teaspoon cayenne pepper (optional for spice)
- 1 can (14 oz) diced tomatoes
- Salt to taste
- Fresh cilantro leaves for garnish
- Cooked rice or naan bread for serving

Instructions:

- After the water runs clean, rinse the red lentils under cold water.
- Boil four cups of water in a big saucepan. Lower the heat and add the rinsed lentils. Cook the lentils for 15 to 20 minutes, covered, or until they are soft and thoroughly cooked. When necessary, add more water and stir periodically.
- Heat the olive oil in a different skillet over medium heat. Add the chopped onion and cook for approximately 5 minutes, or until it softens.
- Fill the skillet with grated ginger and chopped garlic. Cook for a further two minutes, or until aromatic.
- Add the ground coriander, cumin, turmeric, garam masala, and cayenne pepper (if used) and stir. Cook, stirring regularly, for one minute.
- Cook the diced tomatoes in the pan for five minutes, stirring now and again.

- Add the tomato mixture to the lentil pot when the lentils have finished cooking. After thoroughly mixing, add salt to taste.
- To give the flavors time to blend, simmer the lentil dal for a further five to ten minutes.
- Garnish the hot vegan lentil dal with fresh cilantro leaves, drawing inspiration from Indian cuisine. Savor it with naan bread or boiled rice.

17. Moroccan Chickpea Tagine with Couscous:

Ingredients:

- 1 tablespoon olive oil
- 1 onion, chopped
- 3 cloves garlic, minced
- 1 teaspoon ground cumin
- 1 teaspoon ground coriander
- 1 teaspoon paprika

- ½ teaspoon ground cinnamon
- ¼ teaspoon ground ginger
- ¼ teaspoon ground turmeric
- 1 can (15 oz) chickpeas, drained and rinsed
- 1 can (14 oz) diced tomatoes
- 1 cup vegetable broth
- 1 cup diced carrots
- 1 cup diced potatoes
- ½ cup chopped dried apricots
- Salt and pepper to taste
- Cooked couscous for serving
- Chopped fresh cilantro for garnish

Instructions:

- Heat the olive oil in a big pan or tagine over medium heat. Add the chopped onion and cook for approximately 5 minutes, or until it softens.
- Cook the minced garlic in the pan for a further two minutes, or until it becomes fragrant.
- Add the ground turmeric, ground ginger, ground cinnamon, ground coriander,

paprika, and ground cumin. Cook, stirring regularly, for one minute.

- Fill the pan with the diced carrots, diced potatoes, diced tomatoes, chopped dried apricots, and drained chickpeas. To taste, add salt and pepper for seasoning.

- Simmer the mixture for a little while before turning down the heat. Once the flavors have blended and the veggies are soft, simmer them for 20 to 25 minutes while covered.

- Transfer the heated Moroccan chickpea tagine to a bed of prepared couscous. Before serving, add some freshly cut cilantro as a garnish.

Chapter 4

Sample Meal Plans for Each Trimester

- **First Trimester**

Breakfast:
- Overnight oats made with rolled oats, almond milk, chia seeds, and topped with fresh berries and sliced almonds
- Herbal tea or water with lemon

Mid-Morning Snack:
- Sliced apple with almond butter

Lunch:
- Quinoa salad with mixed greens, cherry tomatoes, cucumber, avocado, black beans, and a lemon-tahini dressing
- Whole grain crackers on the side

Afternoon Snack:
- Carrot sticks with hummus

Dinner:
- Baked tofu with roasted sweet potatoes and steamed broccoli
- Side salad with mixed greens, shredded carrots, and balsamic vinaigrette

Evening Snack:
- Vegan yogurt with granola and a sprinkle of ground flaxseeds

- **Second Trimester**

Breakfast:
- Smoothie made with spinach, frozen berries, banana, silken tofu, and almond milk
- Whole grain toast with avocado slices

Mid-Morning Snack:
- Handful of mixed nuts and dried fruits

Lunch:
- Lentil soup with whole grain bread
- Side salad with mixed greens, cherry tomatoes, bell peppers, and a drizzle of olive oil and lemon juice

Afternoon Snack:
- Rice cakes topped with mashed avocado and sliced cucumber

Dinner:
- Stuffed bell peppers filled with quinoa, black beans, corn, and diced tomatoes, topped with vegan cheese and baked until tender
- Steamed green beans on the side

Evening Snack:
- Sliced mango with coconut yogurt and a sprinkle of shredded coconut

- **Third Trimester**

Breakfast:
- Whole grain pancakes topped with sliced bananas, almond butter, and a drizzle of maple syrup
- Green tea or decaffeinated coffee with almond milk

Mid-Morning Snack:
- Homemade trail mix with mixed nuts, seeds, and dried fruits

Lunch:
- Chickpea salad wrap with whole grain tortilla, mixed greens, shredded carrots, cucumber, avocado, and hummus
- Baby carrots and cherry tomatoes on the side

Afternoon Snack:
- Celery sticks filled with peanut butter and raisins (ants on a log)

Dinner:
- Lentil and vegetable stir-fry served over brown rice
- Steamed edamame on the side

Evening Snack:
- Baked sweet potato topped with cinnamon and a dollop of coconut yogurt

Beverage Recipes to Stay Hydrated and Energized

Green Smoothie:

Ingredients:
- 1 cup spinach leaves
- 1 cup kale leaves, stems removed
- 1 ripe banana, peeled
- 1 cup pineapple chunks
- 1 cup coconut water

Instructions:
- Blend together the kale, spinach, banana, pineapple pieces, and coconut water in a blender.
- Process on high speed until creamy and smooth.
- Immediately serve after pouring into glasses.

Citrus Infused Water:

Ingredients:
- 1 lemon, thinly sliced
- 1 lime, thinly sliced
- 1 orange, thinly sliced
- 8 cups water (2 liters)

Instructions:
- Slice the orange, lime, and lemon thinly and place them in a pitcher.
- Drizzle the citrus segments with water.
- Gently mix everything together.
- To enable the flavors to meld, refrigerate for a minimum of one hour.
- Present cold, on top of ice.

Energizing Matcha Latte:

Ingredients:
- 1 teaspoon matcha powder
- ¼ cup hot water
- ¾ cup almond milk (or any plant-based milk of choice)
- Optional: sweetener of choice (such as honey, maple syrup, or stevia)

Instructions:
- Mix the matcha powder and hot water in a cup, whisking until the matcha is completely dissolved.
- Use a pot or microwave to preheat the almond milk until it is warm but not boiling.
- Add the heated almond milk to the matcha concoction and whisk to create foam.
- If desired, sweeten to taste with your favorite sweetener.
- Present right away.

Cucumber Mint Cooler:

Ingredients:
- 1 cucumber, peeled and chopped
- ¼ cup fresh mint leaves
- Juice of 1 lime
- 2 tablespoons honey (or maple syrup for vegan option)
- 4 cups water (1 liter)

Instructions:
- Add the diced cucumber, mint leaves, lime juice, honey, and water to a blender.
- Blend until well mixed and smooth.
- To get rid of any pulp, strain the mixture using a fine-mesh sieve.
- Pour the cucumber-mint cooler into a pitcher and place in the fridge to cool.
- If preferred, top with more mint leaves and serve over ice.

Berry Blast Smoothie:

Ingredients:
- 1 cup mixed berries (such as strawberries, blueberries, raspberries)
- ½ cup Greek yogurt
- 1 cup almond milk
- 1 tablespoon honey (or maple syrup for vegan option)

Instructions:
- Blend together the Greek yogurt, almond milk, honey, and mixed berries using a blender.
- Process on high speed until creamy and smooth.
- Taste and add additional honey if necessary to adjust sweetness.
- Immediately serve after pouring into glasses.

Iced Herbal Tea:

Ingredients:
- 4 herbal tea bags (your choice of flavor)
- 8 cups cold water (2 liters)

Instructions:
- The herbal tea bags should be placed in a big pitcher.
- Cover the tea bags with cold water.
- To let the tea bags soak in the cold water, cover the pitcher and place it in the refrigerator for the whole night.
- Take out the tea bags from the pitcher the next day.
- Top with ice cubes and garnish with mint or lemon, if you'd like, before serving the chilled herbal tea.

Tropical Turmeric Smoothie:

Ingredients:
- 1 cup pineapple chunks
- 1 cup mango chunks
- ½ teaspoon ground turmeric
- 1 teaspoon fresh ginger, grated
- 1 cup coconut water

Instructions:
- Grated ginger, ground turmeric, pineapple and mango pieces, and coconut water should all be combined in a blender.
- Process on high speed until creamy and smooth.
- Taste and add your preferred sweetener to adjust sweetness if necessary.
- Immediately serve after pouring into glasses.

Watermelon Lime Slushie:

Ingredients:
- 4 cups watermelon chunks, seeds removed
- Juice of 2 limes
- 2 cups ice cubes

Instructions:
- Lime juice and watermelon pieces should be combined in a blender.
- Fill the blender with the ice cubes.
- Process the mixture at a high speed until it becomes smooth and slushy.
- Taste and add your preferred sweetener to adjust sweetness if necessary.
- Immediately serve after pouring into glasses.

Energizing Beet Juice:

Ingredients:
- 2 medium-sized beets, peeled and chopped
- 2 large carrots, peeled and chopped
- 2 apples, cored and chopped
- 1-inch piece of fresh ginger, peeled
- Optional: lemon juice or lime juice for added freshness (to taste)

Instructions:
- To extract the juice, run the diced apples, ginger, carrots, and beets through a juicer.
- To improve the taste, stir with lime or lemon juice, if preferred.
- Immediately serve the vivid beet juice by pouring it into glasses.

Chia Seed Fresca:

Ingredients:
- 2 tablespoons chia seeds
- 2 cups water (480 ml)
- Juice of 1 lemon or lime
- 1-2 tablespoons agave syrup or maple syrup, to taste

Instructions:
- The chia seeds and water should be combined in a glass or container. Stir well to avoid clumping.
- Soak the chia seeds in the water for ten to fifteen minutes, stirring now and again, until they take on the consistency of gel.
- Mix the agave syrup and lemon or lime juice into the chia gel. Mix well until fully incorporated.
- To cool and let the flavors combine, place the chia fresca in the refrigerator for a minimum of half an hour.

- Before serving, give the fresca one more stir since the chia seeds could sink to the bottom of the glass.
- If preferred, pour the chia seed fresca over ice cubes into glasses.

Staying active and healthy during pregnancy

It is crucial for the mother's health as well as the baby's best possible growth.

Speak with a Healthcare Professional: To make sure an exercise program is healthy for both the mother and the unborn child, it's crucial to speak with an obstetrician or other healthcare professional before beginning one during pregnancy. Based on each person's unique health situation and demands throughout pregnancy, they may provide tailored advice.

Select Safe and Appropriate Exercises: Go for low-impact, pregnancy-safe activities that are easy on the joints, such swimming, strolling, stationary cycling, prenatal yoga, and water aerobics. Steer clear of activities that put you at risk for falls or injuries to your abdomen, such contact sports, skiing, and intense high-impact aerobics.

Listen to Your Body: Pay attention to the cues that your body gives you and modify your level of activity appropriately. It's crucial to relax and take a break if you feel worn out, lightheaded, or uncomfortable in any other way. Don't overwork yourself; instead, put your comfort and wellbeing first.

Maintain excellent Posture: As the pregnancy goes on, it might become more noticeable how much pressure is placed on the back and joints. To ease this strain, adopt excellent posture. Steer clear of prolonged standing or sitting, and use pillows or supporting cushions as required to provide comfort.

Perform Pelvic Floor Exercises: Also referred to as Kegel exercises, these exercises strengthen the muscles of the pelvic floor and lower the risk of pelvic floor dysfunction and urine incontinence both during and after pregnancy.

Eat a Well-Balanced Diet: To improve general health and energy levels throughout pregnancy, eat a nutritious, well-balanced diet. Eat a lot of fruits, vegetables, whole grains, lean meats, and healthy fats. These foods are high in nutrients.

Get adequate Sleep and Rest: To maintain your physical and emotional health during your pregnancy, make obtaining adequate sleep and rest a priority. Pay attention to your body's demand for relaxation and rest, particularly if you feel like you're more tired than usual throughout pregnancy.

Practice Stress Management: To encourage relaxation and lessen anxiety throughout pregnancy, use stress-relieving practices including deep breathing exercises, meditation, prenatal massage, and relaxation methods.

Take Prenatal Exercise courses: Prenatal fitness instructors with certifications might consider offering prenatal exercise courses or seminars. These courses may provide advice on safe and efficient workouts catered specifically to the requirements of expectant mothers.

Chapter 5

Preparing for Labor and Delivery: Nutrition Tips and Tricks

In addition to being mentally and physically ready, preparing for labor and delivery also include eating a healthy diet to meet the body's demands throughout this life-changing experience.

Remain Hydrated: To keep hydrated and maintain the ideal fluid balance, drink plenty of water throughout the day. During childbirth, dehydration may impair general wellbeing and cause weariness. Try to have eight to ten glasses of water a day, or more if it's hot outside or you're physically active.

Eat Well-Balanced Meals: Make sure your meals are well-balanced by including a range of nutrient-dense foods from every food category. For energy, power, and endurance throughout labor, concentrate on including lean proteins, complex carbs, healthy fats, fruits, and vegetables in your diet.

Consume Foods High in Fiber: Try to include foods high in fiber in your meals, such as fruits, vegetables, whole grains, legumes, and nuts, to help maintain healthy digestive tracts and avoid constipation, which may exacerbate labor pains.

Consume Iron-Rich Foods: To avoid iron deficiency anemia, which may exacerbate weakness and exhaustion during delivery and the postpartum period, make sure you are getting enough iron from foods like leafy greens, lentils, beans, tofu, fortified cereals, and lean meats.

Choose Nutrient-Rich Snacks: To provide enduring energy and stave off hunger throughout labor, have nutrient-rich snacks available. Trail mix, fruit and yogurt, nut butter on whole grain crackers, hummus on veggie sticks, or a fruit and cheese slice are all healthy choices.

Incorporate Foods High in Protein: To promote muscular strength and regeneration throughout birth and recovery, give priority to foods high in protein, such as lean meats, poultry, fish, eggs, dairy products, tofu, tempeh, legumes, and nuts.

Incorporate Omega-3 Fatty Acids: To promote brain health and minimize inflammation during labor, include sources of omega-3 fatty acids in your diet, such as walnuts, hemp seeds, chia seeds, flaxseeds, and fatty fish (like salmon and trout).

Restrict Processed meals and Added Sugars: Try to limit your intake of processed meals, sugar-filled snacks, and drinks since they are high in empty calories and may cause blood sugar swings and energy dumps during labor. Whenever possible, choose whole, minimally processed meals.

Think About Small, Frequent Meals: Eating smaller, more frequent meals or snacks instead of larger ones may help you stay energized and avoid pain as labor draws near. Take heed to your body's signals of hunger and fullness and adjust your diet appropriately.

Remain Adaptable: Since labor is erratic, you may not always feel like eating or have particular dietary needs at this time. Remain adaptable and concentrate on eating palatable, easily digested meals. Don't worry about following a meal plan to the letter.

Discuss with Your Healthcare Provider: To make sure that your food choices are appropriate for your particular health needs and pregnancy status, speak with your healthcare provider or a registered dietitian before making any significant changes to your diet or nutrition plan in preparation for labor.

Postpartum Nutrition for Vegan Moms

For vegan mothers to aid in their recuperation, restore their nutritional reserves, and provide sustenance if they want to nurse, postpartum nutrition is essential.

Give special attention to whole, plant-based foods including fruits, vegetables, whole grains, legumes, nuts, and seeds that are high in vital nutrients. These foods include a variety of vitamins, minerals, fiber, and antioxidants that are essential for general health and postpartum recuperation.

Include enough protein in your meals to aid with muscle recovery, tissue regeneration, and, if necessary, lactation. Tofu, tempeh, legumes (beans, lentils, and chickpeas), quinoa, nuts, seeds, and plant-based protein powders are excellent vegan sources of protein.

Postpartum recuperation needs an increased intake of iron, particularly if blood loss occurred following delivery. To restore iron reserves and avoid iron deficiency anemia, include plant foods high in iron, such as leafy greens, lentils, beans, fortified cereals, tofu, and pumpkin seeds.

These fats are critical for maintaining brain function and may help maintain emotional stability in the postpartum period. Incorporate plant-based sources of omega-3s, such as supplements made from algae and foods like flaxseeds, chia seeds, hemp seeds, and walnuts.

Calcium is necessary for strong bones and the production of milk in nursing mothers. Increase your intake of calcium-rich plant foods including almonds, tahini, fortified orange juice, tofu, tempeh, leafy greens (kale, collard greens), and fortified plant milk.

If you're nursing, particularly throughout the day, make sure you drink plenty of water to keep hydrated. Sufficient fluid intake promotes lactation, facilitates the healing process after childbirth, and averts constipation.

To promote digestive health and fend against constipation, which is a typical occurrence during the postpartum period, include foods high in fiber, such as fruits, vegetables, whole grains, legumes, nuts, and seeds.

To sustain energy levels, control blood sugar, and promote milk production if nursing, try to eat frequently spaced, well-balanced meals and snacks throughout the day. Every meal or snack should have a combination of healthy fats, proteins, and carbs.

Vegan mothers may find it helpful to take supplements including calcium, iron, vitamin B12, vitamin D, and omega-3 fatty acids, depending on their unique nutritional requirements and food consumption. For advice on the proper dose of supplements, speak with a licensed nutritionist or healthcare professional.

Throughout the postpartum phase, don't forget to give relaxation and self-care first priority. During this period, maintaining a healthy diet, drinking enough water, and getting enough sleep are crucial for both mental and physical health.

Conclusion

The "High Protein, Diabetic-Friendly Vegan Pregnancy Cookbook For First-Time Moms" offers a thorough how-to manual for overcoming the special dietary requirements and difficulties associated with a vegan pregnancy. Pregnant women may survive throughout pregnancy and beyond with the information and recipes in this book. From controlling blood sugar levels and knowing the fundamentals of vegan nutrition to cooking tasty and nutritious meals for every trimester and beyond. Expectant mothers who choose a plant-based diet high in protein, crucial nutrients, and flavorful foods may take care of their own health, promote their unborn child's healthy growth, and take on parenthood with vigor and confidence. Cheers to a joyful, healthful, and delectable vegan pregnant experience!

Review

I highly value your opinion and would greatly appreciate it if you could take a moment to share your thoughts on this cookbook. Your feedback is invaluable as it helps me to understand what you enjoyed and how I can further improve. Your review will also assist other potential readers in deciding whether this book is right for them.

Thank you for taking the time to share your thoughts and experience.

Warm Regards,

Bertha Seward

www.ingramcontent.com/pod-product-compliance
Lightning Source LLC
Chambersburg PA
CBHW061629250726
48659CB00004B/1144